Contents

UROGYNAECOLOGY

The
Investigation
and
Management
of
Urinary
Incontinence
in
Women

Edited by
A.R.B. Smith

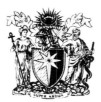

RCOG Press

First published 1995

© Royal College of Obstetricians and Gynaecologists 1995

ISBN 0-902331-66-3

Published by the RCOG Press at the
Royal College of Obstetricians and Gynaecologists
27 Sussex Place, Regent's Park
London NW1 4RG

Registered Charity No. 213280

Cover designed by Geoffrey Wadsley
Printed by Latimer Trend & Co Ltd, Plymouth

Contributors

Professor Linda D. Cardozo
Consultant Obstetrician and Gynaecologist, Kings College Hospital Medical School, Denmark Hill, London SE5 8RX

Dr Alfred S. Cutner
Senior Registrar in Obstetrics and Gynaecology, Farnborough Hospital, Farnborough Common, Orpington, Kent BR6 8ND

Dr Magnus Fall
Associate Professor and Chief Urologist, Department of Surgery, Section of Urology, Sahlgrenska Hospital, Goteborg University, S-413 45 Sweden

Mr Paul Hilton
Consultant Gynaecologist, Subspecialist in Urogynaecology, Royal Victoria Infirmary and Associated Hospitals NHS Trust, Queen Victoria Road, Newcastle upon Tyne NE1 4LP

Mr David Holmes
Lead Consultant Obstetrician and Gynaecologist, St Paul's Hospital, Swindon Road, Cheltenham, Gloucestershire GL50 4BW

Mr Graham James
Director of Business Development and Contracting, Department of Planning and Contracting, Cobbett House, Manchester Royal Infirmary, Oxford Road, Manchester M13 9WL

Mr Gerald J. Jarvis
Consultant Gynaecologist, Department of Urogynaecology, St James's University Hospital, Beckett Street, Leeds LS9 7TF

Dr Vik Khullar
Registrar, Kings College Hospital Medical School, Denmark Hill, London SE5 8RX

Mr Ed Kiff
Consultant Colorectal Surgeon, Withington Hospital, Nell Lane, West Didsbury, Manchester M20 8LE

Dr Jacqueline M. Lavin
WellBeing Training Fellow, Department of Urological Gynaecology, St Mary's Hospital for Women and Children, Whitworth Park, Manchester M13 0JH

Mr William T. Lawrence
Consultant Urologist, Eastbourne District General Hospital, Kings Drive, Eastbourne, East Sussex BN21 2UD

Dr Jo Laycock
Urotherapy Manager, Department of Urotherapy, Bradford Royal Infirmary, Duckworth Lane, Bradford, West Yorkshire BD9 6RJ

Dr Sivert Lindstrom
Department of Cell Biology, University of Health Sciences, Linkoping, Sweden

Sister Jill Lord
Nurse Practitioner, Department of Urogynaecology, St Mary's Hospital for Women and Children, Whitworth Park, Manchester M13 0JH

Mr Ash K. Monga
Senior Registrar, Urogynaecology Unit, St George's Hospital, Blackshaw Road, London SW17 0RE

Dr Kristina Naidoo
Senior Registrar, Stepping Hill Hospital, Poplar Grove, Stockport, Cheshire SK2 7JE

Mr Timothy R. Sayer
Consultant Obstetrician and Gynaecologist, North Hampshire Hospital, Aldermaston Road, Basingstoke, Hampshire RG24 9NA

Mr Julian Shah
Senior Lecturer and Honorary Consultant Urologist, Institute of Urology and Nephrology, 48 Riding House Street, London W1P 7PN

Dr A. R. B. Smith
Consultant Gynaecologist, Department of Urological Gynaecology, St Mary's Hospital for Women and Children, Whitworth Park, Manchester M13 0JH

Mr Clive Spence-Jones
Senior Lecturer, Department of Obstetrics and Gynaecology, St Bartholomew's Hospital, West Smithfield, London EC1A 7BE

Mr Stuart L. Stanton
Consultant Gynaecologist, Urogynaecology Unit, St George's Hospital, Blackshaw Road, London SW17 0RE

Introduction

This book is largely derived from lectures delivered during the RCOG meeting held in London in 1994. The contributors were chosen for their experience in particular areas of interest within the subspecialty so that a balance of general review and personal experience is given.

The paper on the role of the nurse in the investigation and management of incontinence provoked a lively debate at the meeting and reflects a departure from convention. It is possible that the skills many nurses involved with incontinence undoubtedly possess are currently underidentified.

Any subspecialist service must be set up and maintained with good business planning. The paper on purchaser–provider considerations gives an introduction to an area many clinicians find both alien and difficult.

The increasing recognition that urinary and faecal incontinence commonly co-exist led to the inclusion of two papers on ano-rectal incontinence. The association of obstetric events with the development of incontinence means that the obstetrician and gynaecologist should have an understanding of the aetiology, investigation and management of all types of incontinence. This, on occasion, will require close collaboration with urologists and colorectal surgeons.

I am indebted to the authors for their contributions and hope that the book proves interesting and stimulating.

Tony Smith
Manchester 1995

1

Anatomy and physiology of the lower urinary tract and the pathophysiology of urinary incontinence and sensory disorders of the lower urinary tract

Paul Hilton

Introduction

Urinary incontinence may be defined as 'a condition in which involuntary loss of urine is a social or hygienic problem, and is objectively demonstrable'. Continence then, by inference, might be considered as the ability to retain urine within the bladder between voluntary acts of micturition. In order to comprehend the pathological processes which lead to the development of urinary incontinence, a clear understanding of the normal mechanisms for the maintenance of continence is fundamental; this in turn must be based on a knowledge of the morphology and physiology of the bladder and urethra, and their supporting structures.

Anatomy of the lower urinary tract

The bladder

Detrusor

The smooth muscle of the bladder is often described as consisting of three distinct layers, the outer being orientated longitudinally, the middle circularly, and the inner longitudinally. There is, however, frequent interchange of fibres between bundles, and from a functional point of view, the detrusor appears constructed so as to contract as a single syncytial mass. With the exception of the muscle fibres of the superficial trigone, all areas of the detrusor contain significant amounts of acetyl-cholinesterase, in keeping with their abundant cholinergic parasympathetic nerve supply.

Trigone

The smooth muscle of the trigone, in contrast to that of the rest of the bladder is easily distinguished into two distinct layers (see Figure 1.1). The deep trigonal muscle is in all respects similar to the detrusor; the superficial muscle in this region, however,

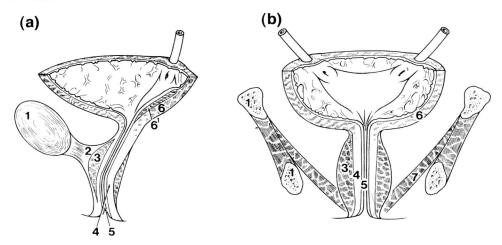

Figure 1.1 Schematic diagrams of female bladder and urethra in sagittal section (a) and coronal section (b). 1. symphysis/rami; 2. posterior pubo-urethral ligaments; 3. intrinsic striated muscle (rhabdosphincter urethrae); 4. intrinsic smooth muscle; 5. mucosa and submucosal vascular tissues; 6. smooth muscle of detrusor/deep trigone; 6^1. smooth muscle of superficial trigone; 7. extrinsic striated muscle/levator ani. (Reproduced from Hilton, P. (1986) 'The mechanism of continence', in: S. L. Stanton and E. A. Tanagho (Eds) *Surgery for Female Incontinence*. London and Berlin: Springer-Verlag. With permission of the author and publisher)

is relatively thick and consists of small muscle bundles; the cells themselves are devoid of acetyl-cholinesterase and have a more sparse cholinergic nerve supply. It is continuous with the ureteric smooth muscle and it has been suggested that it may have significance in the control of the ureterovesical junction during voiding, thereby preventing ureteric reflux.

Bladder neck

The smooth muscle of the bladder neck is also distinct from that of the detrusor. In the male a well-defined pre-prostatic smooth muscle sphincter is present; in the female, however, the orientation of bundles is largely oblique or longitudinal and they appear to have little or no sphincter action.

The urethra

The normal female urethra is between 30 and 50 mm in length from internal to external meatus. Its structure, in particular that of the smooth and striated muscle components, has been the subject of considerable debate.

Urethral smooth muscle

A smooth muscle coat runs throughout the length of the female urethra, in a largely longitudinal direction. Whilst morphologically the smooth muscle of the detrusor and that of the urethra may appear continuous, histochemically they are different in that the urethral smooth muscle cells are devoid of the acetyl-cholinesterase which is found in profusion within the cells of the detrusor. It seems unlikely that this component plays any major active role in continence, since its contraction will result in shortening and widening of the urethra; the inherent elasticity of the tissues may, however, contribute passively to bladder neck closure.

Urethral and periurethral striated muscle

The intrinsic striated portion of the urethral sphincter mechanism (the external sphincter, or rhabdosphincter urethrae) consists of bundles of circularly arranged fibres maximum in bulk at the mid-urethral level anteriorly, thinning laterally, and being almost totally deficient posteriorly (see Figure 1.1). The extrinsic periurethral muscle of levator ani, in contrast, has no direct contiguity with the urethra, being separated from it by a distinct connective tissue septum. It has also been demonstrated that these muscles are histochemically distinct, and of different functional specialisation. The intrinsic striated muscle is made up of small diameter muscle fibres, rich in acid stable myosin ATPase, and possessing numerous mitochondria; they are therefore classified as slow twitch fibres, and are thought to be responsible for the striated muscle contribution to urethral closure at rest. By contrast, the extrinsic periurethral striated muscles are made up of a heterogeneous population of fibres, some of which show the above characteristics of slow twitch muscle, while others are rich in alkaline stable ATPase, characteristic of fast twitch muscle. The latter fibres are suspected to contribute an additional reflex component to aid urethral closure on stress.

Mucosa and submucosa

The epithelial lining of the urethra is of two types; proximally it is continuous with that of the bladder and consists of pseudostratified transitional cells; distally it is continuous with introital skin, and consists of non-keratinised stratified squamous cells. The junction between the two varies with age and oestrogen status and may be of significance with regard to the prevention of ascending infection.

Within the submucosa of the female urethra two prominent venous plexi have been identified; a distal one whose structure varies little with age, and a proximal one beneath the bladder neck, where marked age-related changes are seen. In women of reproductive age the vessels are highly folded, thin walled, and with numerous arterio-venous anastomoses, giving a cavernous appearance to the submucosa not seen in postmenopausal women. These findings have been interpreted as indicating that the urethral vascular system plays a major role in the closure of the urethra in young women.

Urethral supports

The so-called pubo-urethral or pubovesical ligaments are thought to form an important component of the suspensory mechanism for the female bladder neck. In fact these 'ligaments' contain large numbers of smooth muscle bundles, which extend upwards towards the lower fibres of the bladder, and it is possible therefore that they provide both active and passive components to the maintenance of the normal spatial relationships of urethra, bladder and pelvis. More recently DeLancey (1988) has investigated the supports of the urethra, and has described both muscular and fascial attachments of the anterior vaginal wall in the region of the proximal urethra to the arcus tendineus fasciae pelvis, such that contraction of the pelvic diaphragm pulls the vagina against the urethra, creating compression posteriorly. He also described two arches of muscle running over the urethra (the compressor urethrae and the urethro-vaginal sphincter) which compress it distally.

Neurological control of micturition

The main function of the bladder is to convert the continuous excretory process of the kidneys into a more convenient, intermittent process of evacuation. This calls for an extraordinarily complex neural control to coordinate sensory input from, and motor output to, bladder and urethra in reciprocal fashion (see Figure 1.2).

Innervation of the detrusor

Parasympathetic supply

Pre-ganglionic parasympathetic fibres with cell bodies in the intermediolateral grey columns of the sacral segments S_2 to S_4 run in the pelvic splanchnic nerves through the pelvic plexus. Autonomic ganglia are present along the nerve trunks not only within the plexus, but also on its more peripheral branches as they ramify on and within the bladder wall. As a result the bladder muscle is diffusely and richly supplied with cholinergic nerve fibres, to the extent that each individual muscle cell may be supplied by one or more cholinergic nerves.

Sympathetic supply

Pre-ganglionic sympathetic fibres with cell bodies in the intermediolateral grey areas of the thoracic and lumbar segments T_{10} to L_2 travel in the sympathetic chain and then via the lumbar splanchnic nerves to the superior hypogastric plexus. From there the right and left hypogastric nerves ramify within the pelvic plexus.

Noradrenaline, released from the post-ganglionic sympathetic fibres, may be either excitatory or inhibitory depending on the predominant receptor type. Beta receptors, producing relaxation in response to noradrenaline binding, have been shown to predominate in the vault of the bladder, whilst alpha receptor sites, producing contraction, predominate in the bladder base; the significance of the latter in the human female is probably minimal.

Visceral afferent supply

Visceral afferent fibres may be identified travelling with both sacral and thoracolumbar visceral efferent nerves. Sacral afferents have been shown to be evenly distributed between muscle and submucosa throughout the bladder; they appear to convey the sensations of touch, pain, and bladder distension, and are essential to complete normal micturition. Afferents in the thoracolumbar nerves become activated only

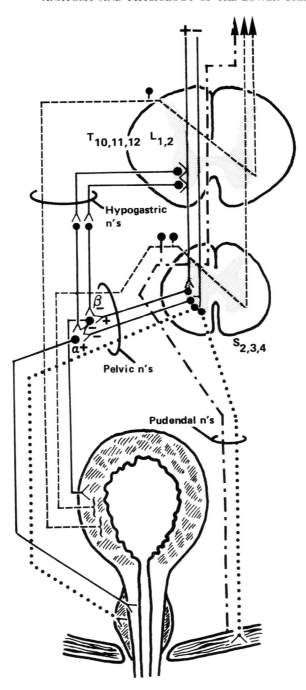

Figure 1.2   Peripheral nerve supply to the lower urinary tract. (———) Visceral efferents (parasympathetic and sympathetic); (————) visceral efferents; (· · · ·) somatic efferents; (— · — ·) somatic efferents. (Reproduced from Hilton, P. (1986) 'The mechanism of continence', in: S. L. Stanton and E. A. Tanagho (Eds) *Surgery for Female Incontinence*. London and Berlin: Springer-Verlag. With permission of the author and publisher)

during marked bladder distension and their transection seems to have little effect on voiding.

Innervation of urethral smooth muscle

Sympathetic and parasympathetic efferent and associated visceral afferent fibres from the vesical plexus also innervate the urethra. Parasympathetic efferents terminate in the urethral smooth muscle, and cholinergic stimulation produces contraction. The orientation of its fibres suggests little sphincteric action, and its parasympathetic innervation suggests importance with respect to voiding function, contraction producing shortening and widening of the urethra along with detrusor contraction during micturition.

Sympathetic efferents also innervate the urethral smooth muscle which possesses predominantly alpha adrenoreceptor sites. Whilst there are no sex differences in adrenergic innervation of the bladder body, the sympathetic innervation of the bladder neck and urethra in the female is much less dense than in the male, where it has been suggested to have a genital rather than urinary function.

Innervation of striated muscle

The innervation of the pelvic floor musculature is important in the assessment and understanding of normal mechanisms of continence, and disorders of both urinary and faecal control. There is still controversy surrounding this area, but there appear to be two embryological components to the pelvic floor, with variations in their innervation. The sphincter cloacae components (the extrinsic periurethral striated muscle, and the external anal sphincter) receive innervation from their perineal aspect, via the pudendal nerves, whereas the pelvi-caudal components (the intramural rhabdosphincter urethrae, and puborectalis muscle) receive innervation from direct motor branches from the pelvic plexus. Both routes of efferent innervation have associated somatic afferent fibres, those from the pelvic floor ascending via the dorsal columns to convey proprioception.

Central nervous connections of the lower urinary tract

The connections of the lower urinary tract within the central nervous system are extraordinarily complex, and many discrete centres with influences on micturition have been identified: within the cerebral cortex, in the superior frontal and anterior cingulate gyri of the frontal lobe, and the paracentral lobule; within the cerebellum, in the anterior vermis and fastigial nucleus, and within subcortical areas including the thalamus, the basal ganglia, the limbic system, the hypothalamus, and discrete areas of the mesencephalic pontine medullary reticular formation.

Cortical centres are important in the perception of sensation from the lower urinary tract and the inhibition and subsequent initiation of voiding. Areas in the superior frontal or anterior cingulate gyri are important in the voluntary control of detrusor function, and that in the paracentral lobule with sphincter function. Lesions of the former are therefore associated with symptoms of urgency and incontinence, and of the latter with urinary retention resulting from spasticity of the pelvic floor.

The thalamus is the principle relay centre for pathways projecting to the cerebral cortex, and ascending pathways activated by bladder and urethral receptors synapse on neurones in specific thalamic nuclei which have been reciprocal connections with the cortex.

Within the pontine reticular formation are two closely related areas with inhibitory and excitatory effects on the sacral micturition centre in the conus medullaris. Lesions of the cord below this always lead to incoordinate voiding with failure of urethral relaxation during detrusor contraction; lesions above this level may be associated with 'normal' though involuntary micturition.

Physiology of the lower urinary tract

Continence is dependent upon the maximum urethral pressure exceeding the bladder pressure, or the 'urethral closure pressure' remaining positive. Normal micturition may be said to result from the controlled reversal of this equilibrium, and incontinence from its uncontrolled reversal. The important aspects of the control of continence therefore are, firstly, those factors which maintain the intravesical pressure low and, secondly, those which ensure that the urethral pressure remains high, or at least higher than intravesical pressure, at all times during the filling and storage phases of the micturition cycle.

The behaviour of the bladder

The tension in the bladder wall itself is in part a passive phenomenon related to the distensibility, or visco-elastic properties of the detrusor, and part an active phenomenon due to the contractility of the muscle and its neurological control.

Properties of the bladder wall

During rapid step-wise filling of the bladder the detrusor pressure rises rapidly, and afterwards decays exponentially with time; this time dependence is similar to that expected of a passive visco-elastic solid. However, under the near static conditions of physiological filling, the detrusor's behaviour is more accurately described as elastic. That is to say, the detrusor pressure rises little as the bladder volume increases from zero to functional capacity (see Figure 1.3).

Contractility of the bladder and its neural control

The neurological control of detrusor contractility is dependent upon a sacral spinal reflex under control of several higher centres as considered earlier in this chapter. This basic reflex arc is best considered as a loop extending from sensory receptors within the bladder wall, through the pelvic plexus and via visceral afferent fibres travelling with the pelvic splanchnic nerves, to enter the spinal cord in the S_2 and S_4 level, via internuncial neurones within the cord synapsing with cell bodies in the intermediolateral grey area of the same sacral levels, and hence via parasympathetic fibres in the pelvic splanchnic nerves through the pelvic plexus to the smooth muscle cells of the detrusor. The stretch receptors or proprioceptors within the bladder wall

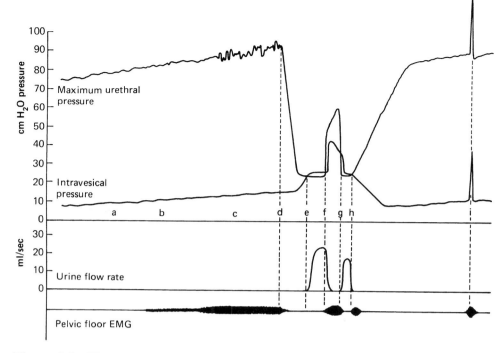

Figure 1.3 The normal micturition cycle showing changes in urethral and intravesical pressure, urine flow rate, and pelvic floor electromyogram.

a. phase of subconscious inhibition;
b. phase of conscious (suppressible) inhibition;
c. phase of reinforced (unsuppressible) inhibition;
d. initiation or transition;
e. voiding;
f. interruption of micturition by pelvic floor contraction;
g. resumption of micturition;
h. end of void;
i. increase in intra-abdominal pressure due to a cough;

(Reproduced from Hilton, P. (1986) 'The mechanism of continence', in: S. L. Stanton and E. A. Tanagho (Eds) *Surgery for Female Incontinence*. London and Berlin: Springer-Verlag. With permission of the author and publisher)

are in effect connected in series with muscle cells and are therefore stimulated by both passive stretch and by active contraction of the detrusor. Once a critical level of stretch is achieved impulses pass in the afferent limb of the reflex arc, and the resultant efferent discharge leads to a detrusor contraction.

The higher control over the basic visceral reflex arc is mediated through descending pathways from the pontine reticular formation. Although both excitatory and inhibitory centres have been located in this region, their net effect is primarily an inhibitory one, and their influence is therefore to prevent contraction of the detrusor, and thus to encourage the maintenance of a low intravesical pressure, during the filling phase of the micturition cycle.

The urethra

In order to maintain continence it is vital not only that the intravesical pressure remains low during the storage phase of the micturition cycle, but also that the urethral lumen should seal completely. Three components of urethral function are necessary to achieve this hermetic property:

1 urethral inner wall softness
2 inner urethral compression
3 outer wall tension.

Whilst the closure of any elastic tube can be obtained if sufficient compression is applied to it, the efficiency of closure is dramatically increased if its lining possesses the property of plasticity, or the ability to mould into a watertight seal.

There has been much debate over the morphological components which contribute to the functional characteristics of softness, compression and tension in the urethra. There is no doubt that the vascularity of the urethra far exceeds the requirements of a blood supply for the organ, and a significant vascular contribution to urethral closure has been suggested. Whatever the contribution of the urethral blood supply to the measured intraluminal pressure, it is likely to be of significance as regards the plasticity of the urothelium and submucosa.

The structures leading to inner wall compression by virtue of their contribution to outer wall tension may include the intramural elastic fibres, the intrinsic smooth and striated muscle, and the extrinsic or periurethral striated muscle. From urethral pressure studies it seems that approximately one third of the resting urethral pressure is due to striated muscle effects, one third to smooth muscle effects, and one third to its vascular supply.

The usual level of continence in the female is not as one might expect, at the level of maximum resting pressure, in the mid-urethra, but at the bladder neck. This region in the female has no sphincteric circular smooth muscle, and is virtually devoid of striated muscle; it would therefore seem that the passive elastic tension is the most important factor leading to closure at the bladder neck level. In mid-urethra the most prominent structural feature is the intrinsic striated muscle or rhabdosphincter, and it is likely that this is responsible for the bulk of active urethral tone at rest. The periurethral striated muscles, in contrast, probably do not contribute greatly to the maintenance of continence at rest but play a significant role in the maintenance of urethral closure in the face of increased intra-abdominal pressure (see 'The mechanism of stress incontinence' later in this Chapter).

The normal micturition cycle

From the background information contained in previous sections of this chapter it is now possible to discuss the mechanisms whereby urine is retained within the bladder during the filling and storage phases, and is evacuated during the voiding phase of the normal micturition cycle (see Figure 1.3).

Filling and storage phase

The bladder normally fills with urine by a series of peristaltic, ureteric contractions, at a rate of between 0.5 and 5 ml/min; under these conditions the bladder pressure increases only minimally. Even during the course of cystometry at rapid filling rates, in normal individuals the pressure rises by no more than $15\,cmH_2O$ from empty to cystometric capacity. Urethral closure meanwhile is maintained by the combined passive and active effects of its smooth and striated muscle components, its elastic content, and its blood supply. The hermetic efficiency is accentuated by the softness of its mucosa.

During the early stages of bladder filling, proprioceptive afferent impulses from stretch receptors within the bladder wall pass via the pelvic nerves to sacral dorsal roots S_2–S_4. These impulses ascend in the cord via the lateral spinothalamic tracts and a detrusor motor response is subconsciously inhibited by descending impulses from the subcortical micturition centres.

As the bladder volume increases, further afferent impulses ascend to the cerebral cortex, and the sensation of bladder filling associated with the desire to micturate is first consciously appreciated, usually at between 200 and 300 ml, or half the functional bladder capacity. The inhibition of detrusor contraction is now cortically mediated, although the desire to void may be further suppressed to subconscious levels again, given sufficient distracting afferent stimuli. With further filling, impulses within the visceral afferent fibres accompanying the sympathetic efferents to thoracolumbar roots T_{10} to L_2 ascend to the cerebral cortex, and a further desire to void is appreciated. During this time, in addition to the cortical suppression of detrusor activity, there may also be a voluntary pelvic floor contraction in an attempt to maintain urethral closure.

Initiation phase

When a suitable time, site and posture for micturition are selected the process of voiding commences. This may be considered in two phases: the initiation, or transition from the non-voiding state, and micturition itself.

Relaxation of the pelvic floor may be shown to occur early in the process, both radiologically and electromyographically; it is likely that simultaneous relaxation of the intrinsic striated muscle also occurs, since a marked fall in intra-urethral pressure is seen before the intravesical pressure rises, during both voluntary and provoked voiding.

A few seconds later the descending inhibitory influences from the cerebral cortex acting on the sacral micturition centre are suppressed, allowing a rapid discharge of efferent parasympathetic impulses via the pelvic nerves, to cause contraction of the detrusor. Depending on the relationship between the force of detrusor contraction and the residual urethral resistance, the intravesical pressure may rise to a variable extent (usually less than $60\,cmH_2O$). When the falling urethral and increasing intravesical pressure equate, urine flow will commence.

Voiding phase

Since the bladder at the initiation of micturition takes on a nearly spherical shape, and has walls which are thin in comparison to its radius, its behaviour may be usefully expressed by the law of Laplace ($P = 2T/R$). As the mural tension rises in the absence of voiding the intravesical pressure also rises. When a critical opening pressure is achieved, urine will start to flow and the bladder radius will fall. The pressure, however, usually remains constant during voiding, and the mural tension therefore must fall. Once initiated, therefore, the process of micturition requires little to sustain it. Whilst active tension is required throughout, the effectiveness of detrusor contraction increases as the muscle fibres shorten and therefore decreasing forces are required as micturition proceeds.

If micturition is voluntarily interrupted midstream, this is usually achieved by a contraction of the periurethral striated muscle of the pelvic floor. In association with this contraction the urethral pressure rises rapidly to exceed the intravesical pressure and therefore urine flow stops. The detrusor, being a smooth muscle, is much slower to relax, and therefore goes on contracting against the closed sphincter. That is to say, an isometric contraction occurs, and again applying the law of Laplace, the intravesical pressure rises. If micturition is resumed by relaxation of the pelvic floor, both urethral and intravesical pressures will return to their previous voiding state.

The mechanism of stress incontinence

The above discussion of the normal micturition cycle relates to the events occurring in a patient essentially at rest, and assumes that intravesical pressure is unaffected by extravesical influences. Acute intra-abdominal pressure rises due to coughing bring at least two additional influences to bear on the mechanisms of continence.

Firstly, there is a passive or direct mechanical transmission of the intra-abdominal pressure increase to the proximal urethra. This effect is dependent upon the normal spatial relationships between the bladder and urethra, and on their fixation in a retropubic position by the posterior pubo-urethral ligaments (see Figure 1.4).

Secondly, it is suggested that a reflex pelvic floor contraction occurs in response to increases in intra-abdominal pressure, which augments urethral closure. Observed pressure changes fit closely with the current concepts of the anatomy of the region, and an active neuromuscular element to the maintenance of normal stress continence is accepted by many authors.

Pathophysiology of urinary incontinence

General considerations

The pathophysiology of several causes of incontinence is considered in greater detail in this volume in chapters relating to individual conditions; here only general comments are made in so far as the pathophysiology relates to abnormalities of the micturition cycle as described above.

Assuming an intact lower urinary tract, urine flow occurs only when the intravesical pressure exceeds the maximum urethral pressure, or when the maximum urethral closure pressure becomes zero or negative. In general terms this may occur as a result of:

1 a fall in urethral pressure associated with an increase in intravesical pressure – as in normal voiding or in many cases of detrusor instability, primarily those of idiopathic or psychosomatic origin, or those resulting from neurological lesions above the level of the pontine micturition centre;

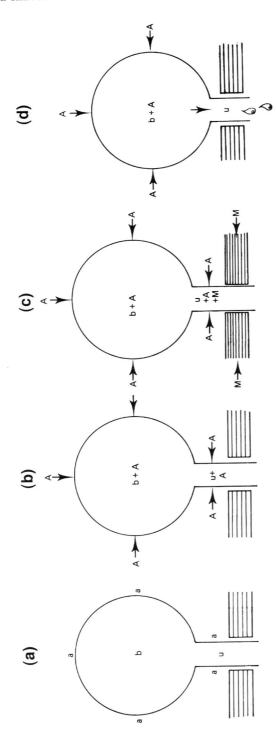

Figure 1.4   Diagram to show the relationship between bladder, urethra, and pelvic floor in the resting state (a) and on stress, to illustrate the passive (b) and active (c) components of pressure transmission to the proximal urethra aiding stress continence. When these components are ineffective stress incontinence results (d). a = resting abdominal pressure; b = resting bladder pressure; u = resting urethral pressure; A = abdominal pressure rise on coughing; M = pelvic floor muscle response on coughing. (Reproduced from Hilton, P. (1987) 'Surgery for urinary stress incontinence', in: J. Monaghan (Ed.) *Operative Surgery: Gynaecology and Obstetrics* (4th ed.). London: Butterworth. With permission of the author and publisher)

2 an increase in intravesical pressure associated with an increase in urethral pressure, the latter being insufficient to maintain a positive closure pressure – as in detrusor instability with associated detrusor sphincter dyssynergia, resulting from neurological lesions above the sacral, but below the pontine micturition centre;

3 an abnormally high increase in detrusor pressure during bladder filling – a situation considered by some workers to be analogous to detrusor instability, but perhaps better considered as impaired bladder compliance; this may be seen in chronic inflammatory conditions such as tuberculosis or interstitial cystitis and also following pelvic irradiation; a similar situation also accounts for the incontinence in chronic urinary retention, where the bladder pressure rises acutely at the end of filling;

4 where there is a sudden profound loss of urethral pressure alone, without any coincident change in intravesical pressure – as in urethral instability, a recently recognised, and uncommon cause of incontinence;

5 where on stress the intravesical pressure rises to a greater extent than the intra-urethral pressure, due to a failure of pressure transmission – as in genuine stress incontinence, the commonest cause of incontinence in the female. The cause of this transmission failure remains controversial, although it seems likely that there are both connective tissue and neuromuscular defects contributing to the problem to a greater or lesser degree in most patients. Denervation injury to the pelvic floor and striated urethral sphincter is known to occur following childbirth, and is found to a greater extent in those with stress incontinence. This may lead to a failure or inefficiency of the active pelvic floor contraction in response to increases in intra-abdominal pressure noted above. Fascial defects are also recognised in stress-incontinent women, not simply affecting the endopelvic fascia and pubo-urethral ligaments, but often in a generalised way; this may contribute to failure of the passive pressure transmission from the abdomen.

Sensory disorders of the lower urinary tract

Sensory disorders are among the most distressing conditions affecting the lower urinary tract; whilst incontinence may be embarrassing and inconvenient, it is rarely painful; abnormalities of bladder sensation may, however, mean that the patient's life is constantly dominated by her bladder. They represent, however, a considerable variety of conditions, with a spectrum of symptomatology, of varying and often uncertain aetiology.

Symptoms and causes

The symptoms characterising these conditions include frequency, nocturia, urgency, dysuria, bladder pain and urethral pain. The main conditions to be considered in the differential diagnosis in patients presenting with such symptoms include:

Infective cystitis and urethritis (including TB and fastidious organisms)
Chemical or radiation cystitis
Bladder stones
Bladder and urethral diverticulae
Transitional cell carcinoma and CIS

Detrusor instability
Uro-genital atrophy
Vulvo-vaginal conditions
Endometriosis
Hypersensitive bladder
Urethral syndrome
Interstitial cystitis

Only the last three of these conditions are given specific consideration here, since they are of uncertain aetiology and pathophysiology, and represent to a greater or lesser extent diagnoses based on symptomatology and the exclusion of other conditions.

Hypersensitive bladder (sensory urgency)

The condition of bladder hypersensitivity, or sensory urgency, is strictly speaking a urodynamic diagnosis, made in patients with frequency and urgency (rarely urge incontinence), in whom the first sensation of filling occurs abnormally early (< 25% of cystometric capacity, or <100 ml), yet who do not demonstrate uninhibited detrusor contractions during provocative cystometry. In some cases this may be no more than a failure of the investigative technique, and such patients may have unstable contractions during their usual daily activities, or indeed demonstrate them during long-term ambulatory monitoring. Such patients have been shown to respond well to bladder retraining, and may be no more than a variant of instability with relatively good detrusor control. The early bladder sensation in the absence of contractions may, however, indicate an as yet poorly defined pathology of afferent innervation.

Urethral syndrome

The urethral syndrome is characterised by the symptom complex of recurrent episodes of frequency (and often urgency) with dysuria, in the absence of urinary infection. It is probably much more prevalent than is commonly recognised, and in one study 40% of women with presumed urinary tract infection (UTI) had repeatedly negative urine cultures. Several aetiologies have been suggested for the condition, including: infection by fastidious organisms, evading identification by standard culture techniques; chemical urethritis; subclinical outflow obstruction or external sphincter spasm; peripheral neuralgia; and psychological factors. Little clear evidence exists for any of these, short of anecdotal response to empirical treatments.

Interstitial cystitis

The label of interstitial cystitis is applied widely, and often inappropriately, to any patient with sensory symptoms in whom urine cultures are negative, and where inflammatory changes are evident at cystoscopy. It is, however, more appropriate to restrict use of the term to those with bladder pain amongst their symptoms, in whom the other diagnoses above have been adequately excluded, who show the characteristic features on cystoscopy. These endoscopic findings include bleeding from the mucosa after an initial filling, with petechiae and glomerulations seen at a subsequent fill, with mucosal splitting or ulceration evident most often over the dome. Deep biopsies usually demonstrate increased numbers of mast cells in the detrusor muscle (>20 cells mm^{-2}).

The aetiology of interstitial cystitis, like that of the 'painful bladder syndrome' (a similar symptom complex, but with normal cystoscopy) remains unclear. Possible aetiologies include allergic phenomena, auto immune processes, disruption of the glycosaminoglycans (GAG) protective layer of the urothelium, undetected infection with fastidious organisms, and a reflex sympathetic dystrophy of the bladder.

Conclusions

If dysfunction of the urinary tract is to be effectively managed, the choice of treatment employed must be optimal. This choice must be based on the firm knowledge of the normal structure and function of the system, and of the mechanisms whereby normal control may break down. Only in the light of this knowledge can the meaningful investigation of the individual patient be carried out. In the case of sensory disorders, much of this background information is lacking, rational treatment thus often eludes us, and management revolves around symptomatic relief. For incontinence, however, this information is largely known, and rational and specific therapy is therefore available for most incontinent patients.

Reference

DeLancey, J.O. (1988) Structural aspects of the extrinsic continence mechanism. *Am J Obstet Gynecol* **72**, 296–301

Suggested reading

Definitions and terminology

Abrams, P.H., Blaivas, J.G., Stanton, S.L. and Andersen, J.T. (1990) Standardisation of terminology of lower urinary tract function. *Br J Obstet Gynaecol* **97** (suppl. no. 6): 1–16

Anatomy of the lower urinary tract

DeLancey, J.O. (1988) Structural aspects of the extrinsic continence mechanism. *Am J Obstet Gynecol* **72**, 296–301
Gosling, J.A., Dixon, J. and Humpherson, J.R. (1983) *Functional Anatomy of the Urinary Tract.* Edinburgh: Churchill-Livingstone
Huisman, A.B. (1983) 'Aspects on the anatomy of the female urethra with special relation to urinary continence' in: U. Ulmsten, (Ed.) *Contributions to Gynaecology and Obstetrics,* vol. 10: *Female Stress Incontinence.* Basel: Karger

Neurological control of micturition

Bradley, W.E., Timm, T.W. and Scott, F.B. (1974) Innervation of the detrusor muscle and urethra. *Urol Clin North Am* **1**, 3–27

Fletcher, T.F. and Bradley, W.E. (1978) Neuroanatomy of the bladder-urethra. *J Urol* **119**, 153–60

Torrens, M. (1990) 'Neurophysiology' in: S.L. Stanton (Ed.) *Clinical Gynaecological Urology* (2nd ed.). Edinburgh: Churchill-Livingstone

Physiology of the lower urinary tract

Rud, T. (1980) The urethral pressure profile in continent women from childhood to old age. *Acta Obstet Gynecol Scand* **59**, 331–5

Rud, T., Anderson, K.E., Asmussen, M. *et al.* (1980) Factors maintaining the intraurethral pressure in women. *Invest Urol* **17**, 343–7

Wein, A. (1986) Physiology of micturition. *Clin Geriat Med* **2**, 689–99

The mechanics and hydrodynamics of bladder and urethra

Griffiths, D.J. (1980) *Urodynamics.* Bristol: Adam Hilger

Hilton, P. (1990) 'Urethral pressure profilometry in the female' in N. George, P. O'Reilly and A. Weiss (Eds) *Diagnostic Techniques in Urology.* London: Grune & Stratton

Zinner, N.R., Ritter, R.C. and Sterling, A.M. (1976) 'The mechanism of micturition' in D.I. Williams and G.D. Chisholm (Eds) *Scientific Foundations of Urology*, pp. 36–51. London: Heinemann

Pathophysiology of urinary incontinence

Anderson, R.S. (1984) A neurogenic element to urinary genuine stress incontinence. *Br J Obstet Gynaecol* **91**, 41–6

Enhorning, G.E. (1961) Simultaneous recording of the intravesical and intraurethral pressure. *Acta Chir Scand* (suppl.) **276**, 1–68

Hilton, P. and Stanton, S.L. (1983) Urethral pressure by microtransducer: the results in symptom-free women and in those with genuine stress incontinence. *Br J Obstet Gynaecol* **90**, 919–33

Smith, A.R.B. (1989) The role of partial denervation of the pelvic floor in the aetiology of genitourinary prolapse and stress incontinence of urine. A neurophysiological study. *Br J Obstet Gynaecol* **96**, 24–8

Smith, A.R.B. (1989) The role of pudendal nerve damage in the aetiology of stress incontinence in women. *Br J Obstet Gynaecol* **96**, 29–32

Sensory disorders of the lower urinary tract

George, N.J.R. and Gosling, J.R. (Eds) *Sensory Disorders of the Bladder and Urethra.* New York: Springer-Verlag

Hanno, P.M., Saskin, D.R., Krane, R.J. and Wein, J. (Eds) (1990) *Interstitial Cystitis.* New York: Springer-Verlag

2

The bladder in pregnancy and the puerperium

Alfred Cutner

The earliest report of changes in the lower urinary tract as a result of pregnancy and labour was from sagittal dissections of two women, one who died in late pregnancy and the other in late labour. This study was followed by subjective assessments and radiological investigations of the lower urinary tract in pregnancy. The advent of urodynamic investigations and electromyography has resulted in a better understanding of normal and abnormal function of the lower urinary tract both in pregnancy and in the puerperium. Long-term sequelae have also been assessed by studies performed some time interval after pregnancy and various inferences drawn.

Although urinary tract infections, calculi and fistulae occur coincidental and as a result of pregnancy, this chapter will concentrate on genuine stress incontinence, detrusor instability and voiding difficulties and their related symptomatology.

Symptoms

Lower urinary tract symptoms are very common in pregnancy. To date most studies have been concerned with the prevalence of abnormal voiding patterns and stress incontinence. More recently other symptoms such as urgency, urge incontinence, and symptoms of voiding difficulties have been explored.

Voiding patterns

There are no standardised definitions of voiding patterns and most studies are not comparable due to differing definitions. Early reports suggested that diurnal frequency occurred in about 50% of women in the first trimester and speculated that during this time it was due to pressure on the bladder and thereafter due to recurrent urinary residuals often accompanied by infection. Francis (1960) questioned 400 women personally and found that the onset of frequency usually occurred in the first trimester but once present it tended to get worse and did not resolve as was previously thought (Table 2.1). In addition she found that 81% of women experienced frequency of micturition at some stage in pregnancy and that the prevalence was the same in both nulliparous and multiparous women. The later study of Stanton

17

Table 2.1   The prevalence of frequency in pregnancy according to Francis (1960)

Early pregnancy (%)	Mid pregnancy (%)	Late pregnancy (%)
59.5	61	81

Table 2.2   The prevalence of frequency according to Stanton *et al.* (1980)

	Before pregnancy	Booking	32/40	36/40	38/40	40/40	Postnatal
				%			
Day	16	45	61	72	76	85	17
Night	4	22	37	46	57	64	6
Combined	1	12	27	32	43	54	1

et al. (1980) (Table 2.2) largely agreed with Francis, although it used different definitions.

We used the same definitions as Stanton and colleagues and found a similar prevalence of frequency (43%), nocturia (34%) and combined frequency and nocturia (18%) in early pregnancy (Cutner 1993). Although abnormal voiding patterns appear to be very common in pregnancy and worsen as pregnancy progresses, it is an increase in the actual number of voids which a patient will complain of and in our study 91% of women complained of an increase in the number of voids in a 24-hour period. Furthermore, black women complained of less frequency and more nocturia than their white counterparts and this may further explain differences between previous studies where race was not taken into account.

In ongoing pregnancy we questioned 119 women prior to pregnancy (retrospectively) and at 20 weeks', 28 weeks' and 36 weeks' gestation and postpartum (prospectively) about voiding patterns (Cutner 1993). Figure 2.1 demonstrates the prevalence of frequency and nocturia at each visit. Differences between each visit are significant except between 20 weeks' and 28 weeks' gestation. In addition the prevalence is significantly greater postpartum than prior to pregnancy. Those women who suffered a greater increase in their voiding patterns both during the day and at night were significantly less likely to return to their pre-pregnancy state. This may suggest that abnormal voiding is a learnt phenomenon.

Causes

Early radiological studies in pregnancy found distortion of the fundus of the bladder by the enlarged uterus and suggested that this pressure was likely to result in urinary frequency. However, Francis (1960) carried out radiological visualisation in 83 pregnant women and confirmed distortion of the fundus of the bladder due to the gravid uterus, but she rejected the idea of pressure leading to increased voiding patterns, as it would not explain the high prevalence of nocturia as pressure would be relieved in the recumbent position. In addition, Francis studied urine output in

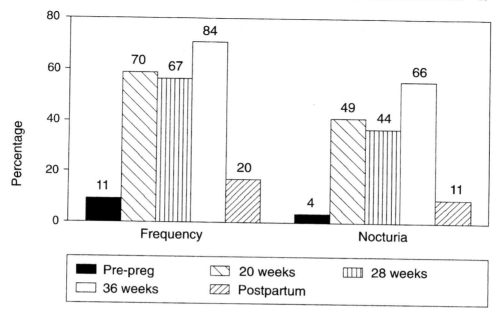

Figure 2.1 Prevalence of frequency and nocturia according to gestation (Cutner 1993)

a series of women in each trimester of pregnancy and concluded that the increased fluid intake and urine output alone was sufficient to explain the prevalence of frequency in pregnancy.

In addition, Parboosingh and Doig (1973) suggested that with regard to nocturia, it is increased sodium excretion at night which results in increased urine production at night. This increased urine production in the first and second trimester would explain the prevalence of nocturia. In the third trimester urine production was reduced. However, the authors found a reduction in the volume of the first morning void and suggest that this would account for the high prevalence of nocturia in the third trimester despite the reduction in urine production.

We studied women in early pregnancy and in ongoing pregnancy and found a significant correlation between the number of voids and urine output. In addition, our results suggest that nocturia may be a result of more hours spent in bed and a decreased functional bladder capacity. Although we found little correlation between lower urinary tract symptoms and urodynamic findings in pregnancy, we did find that women with low compliance had a significantly altered first desire to void and bladder capacity (Cutner 1993) (Table 2.3).

The cystometric capacity of the pregnant bladder has been assessed by several authors. Initial studies found that the bladder capacity gradually increased with increasing gestation but returned to normal by six weeks postpartum. Francis (1960) disputed these findings and found a reduced bladder capacity in the third trimester and no evidence of bladder hypotonia but rather evidence of increased detrusor instability in late pregnancy with unstable detrusor contractions.

Although these studies are contradictory, most of the data are cross-sectional and the relative change rather than absolute values may be of importance. It may be that a combination of pressure effects, altered urine production and a relative change

Table 2.3 First sensation and bladder capacity according to urodynamic diagnosis. Median values given with inter-quartile ranges below. Only significant differences are shown (Cutner 1993)

Parameter	Normal	Low compliance	Phasic DI
First sensation ml	180 150–250 (n = 34)	150 100–150 (n = 23)	160 100–250 (n = 18)
	[p<0.05]		
Bladder capacity ml	420 400–475 (n = 34)	400 300–450 (n = 23)	450 350–500 (n = 18)
	[p<0.05]		[p<0.05]

in bladder capacity leads to the development of frequency and nocturia. However, it is likely that large individual variations make most of the studies to date unreliable.

Prevention and treatment

If the causes are those postulated, then there is no treatment in pregnancy and the patient who is troubled merely needs reassurance. However, if there is a marked increase in these symptoms antenatally or failure for symptoms to resolve postpartum, then she should be investigated for the presence of a lower urinary tract infection. In addition, we have demonstrated (Cutner 1993) that those women who suffer a marked increase in their voiding pattern in pregnancy are less likely to return to their pre-pregnancy state. It would be interesting to determine whether bladder drill antenatally would improve postnatal symptoms in this group of women.

Stress incontinence and urge incontinence

There is much debate as to whether pregnancy itself or labour results in stress incontinence. Although there have been several retrospective and a few prospective studies looking at this subject, it is important to appreciate that stress incontinence is merely a symptom and not synonymous with urethral sphincter incompetence.

Stanton *et al.* (1980) looked at the prevalence of stress incontinence in 181 women and in agreement with earlier studies found that it rarely occurs for the first time postnatally. The prevalence for nulliparous, multiparous and all women is shown in Table 2.4. Analysis of their figures using a Fishers two-tailed test reveals only a significant difference for parity before pregnancy and at the booking visit.

We looked at a multitude of lower urinary tract symptoms in early pregnancy both via direct questioning and visual analogue scores (Figure 2.2). There was a similar prevalence of stress incontinence via both methods of questioning to Stanton *et al.* (1980) but there was also a significant difference in the prevalence of this symptom between white nulliparous and white multiparous women. The same

Table 2.4   Prevalence of stress incontinence according to Stanton *et al.* (1980)

	Before pregnancy	*Booking*	*32/40*	*36/40*	*38/40*	*40/40*	*Post-natal*
				%			
Nulliparous	0	6	30	35	39	34	6
Multiparous	10	27	41	42	41	38	11
Combined	6	17	36	39	40	36	8

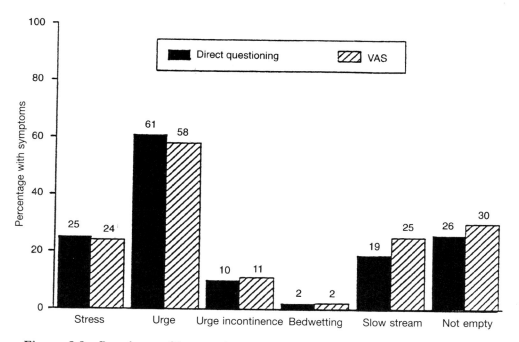

Figure 2.2   Prevalence of lower urinary tract symptoms in early pregnancy on direct questioning and visual analogue scores (VAS) according to Cutner (1993)

symptoms were asked about at several stages of pregnancy in 119 women (Cutner 1993) and the prevalence on direct questioning can be seen in Figure 2.3. Again, results for stress incontinence are similar to those of Stanton and colleagues.

These studies demonstrate a relatively high prevalence of stress incontinence in relation to pregnancy. They suggest that most cases are reversible with only a small minority remaining incontinent long term and that very few cases originate following delivery.

Stanton *et al.* (1980) examined the prevalence of urge incontinence and hesitancy in pregnancy. Urge incontinence reached a peak prevalence of 19% in multiparous

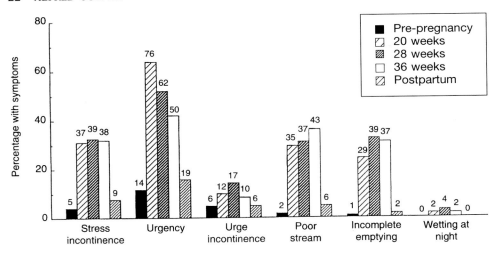

Figure 2.3   Prevalence of lower urinary tract symptoms in pregnancy on direct questioning according to Cutner (1993). Actual numbers are shown above each bar

women. Figures 2.2 and 2.3 demonstrate the prevalence of urgency and urge incontinence in our studies (Cutner 1993). Although these studies suggest the possibility of detrusor instability, again symptoms do not correlate with urodynamic diagnoses. We also found that those women with severe symptoms in pregnancy are more likely to be affected after delivery.

Causes

From the relatively few studies which have looked at lower urinary tract symptoms in pregnancy, it is obvious that functional changes must have occurred. However, it is well known that symptomatology and function correlate poorly in non-pregnant women. Indeed, this lack of agreement has been confirmed in pregnancy (Cutner 1993).

Early radiological studies in pregnancy found changes in the urethro-vesical junction (Malpas *et al.* 1949) (Figure 2.4). In late pregnancy the urethra joined the bladder at right angles but in labour the bladder base was lifted upwards, giving the impression that the urethra was elongated. In women who were examined postnatally the anatomy had returned to normal. These changes in the position of the bladder neck suggest that stretching of supporting structures as a result of labour may lead to damage and weakening of the sphincter mechanisms. Indeed, it has been shown that pregnant fascia has a reduced tensile strength (Landon *et al.* 1990) which may account for the development of stress incontinence in pregnancy. Although postpartum the fascia will regain its previous strength, it may be that in cases of permanent stress incontinence it has already undergone irreversible damage by overstretching.

Anatomical studies do not explain the high prevalence of stress incontinence antenatally with recovery in most cases postpartum. A few studies have examined the lower urinary tract by means of urethral pressure profilometry. Iosif and colleagues assessed 14 women without stress incontinence (Iosif *et al.* 1980) and 12 with stress

Late pregnancy

Early labour

Second stage of labour

After delivery

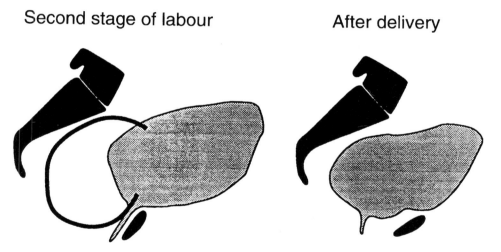

Figure 2.4   Movements of the bladder in labour (modified from Malpas *et al.* 1949)

incontinence (Iosif and Ulmsten 1981) during pregnancy and postpartum. In the continent women there were progressive increases in maximum urethral closure pressure, maximum urethral pressure, functional urethral length and urethral length, with increasing gestation. Postpartum these parameters returned to their early pregnancy values. The increases in maximum urethral closure pressure and functional urethral length were not apparent in the incontinent group and in addition most parameters were significantly reduced compared to the continent group (Figure 2.5). In both groups there was an increase in bladder pressure with progression of pregnancy, and they concluded that these increases in urethral parameters are necessary to maintain continence because of the raised bladder pressures which occur in pregnancy.

Van Geelan et al. (1982) repeated similar work in 43 pregnant women. They failed to show increases in the maximum urethral closure pressure or functional urethral length with increasing gestation. However, they did not divide women into those with and those without stress incontinence and this may have led to different results.

It is important to realise that none of these papers examined the transmission of intra-abdominal pressure to the urethra. There are, however, two reports on the effects of pregnancy on pressure transmission ratios in the French literature which concluded that there was hypertransmission in the first trimester of pregnancy and that increasing parity leads to a cumulative reduction in pressure transmission. Furthermore, they suggested that obstetric trauma in multiparous women may lead to far worse deterioration in urethral function than similar events in first pregnancies.

We compared urethral pressure profile parameters in early pregnancy between those women with and without the symptom of stress incontinence (Cutner 1993) (Figure 2.6). With regard to the maximum urethral closure pressure and maximum urethral pressure, our findings are in agreement with Iosif and colleagues (Iosif et al. 1980, Iosif and Ulmsten 1981). In addition, we found significant differences in pressure transmission ratios. There were also differences in parameters between black and white women (Figure 2.7). This is consistent with the fact that black women suffer genuine stress incontinence to a lesser degree than white women at all ages. When we looked at women during pregnancy and followed them up postpartum, we found the functional urethral length and anatomical urethral length to be significantly greater in pregnancy. It is possible that increased functional urethral length in pregnancy results in improved pressure transmission to the proximal urethra preventing the leakage of urine on stress. However, it must be remembered that the symptom of stress incontinence is taken to signify genuine stress incontinence although the diagnosis of this condition had not been determined by any objective urodynamic criteria.

Electromyography has been used to examine the effects of vaginal delivery on denervation of the sphincter mechanism. It appears that pelvic floor denervation occurs in women who have a vaginal delivery but not in those undergoing a Caesarean section. In addition, the only factor in labour that is associated with severe sphincter damage is a long, active (pushing) second stage (Allen et al. 1990).

Beneficial effects of epidural analgesia have been demonstrated by Dimpfl et al. (1992). They found a lower prevalence of stress incontinence in women who had a forceps delivery under epidural analgesia compared to a pudendal block. Perhaps an epidural affords protection by enabling relaxation of the pelvic floor at the time of delivery.

Our symptom data demonstrated that those women affected badly with stress incontinence at the end of pregnancy are more likely to be affected postnatally (Cutner 1993). We also found that those women with a long first stage of labour were more likely to suffer from this symptom postnatally. There was no correlation with the length of the second stage.

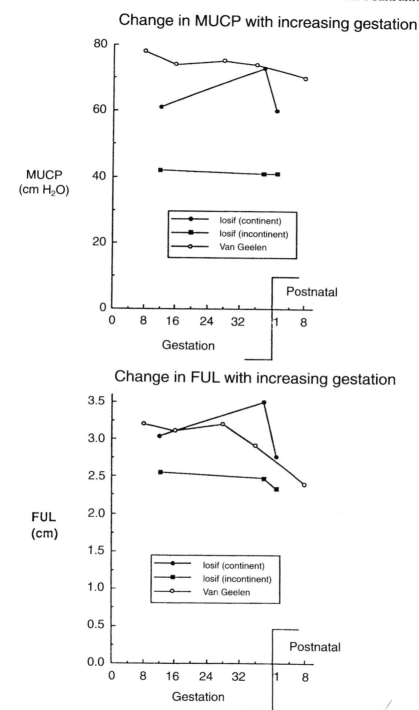

Figure 2.5   Changes in the maximum urethral closure pressure (MUCP) and functional urethral length (FUL) as pregnancy progresses

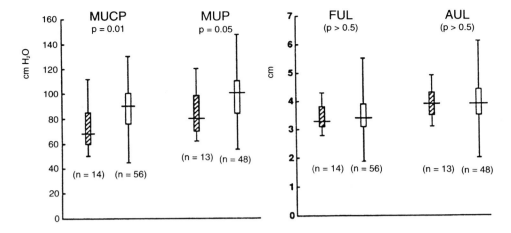

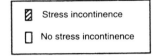

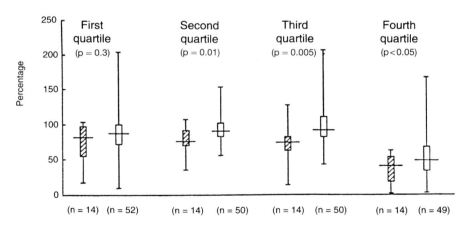

Figure 2.6   Urethral pressure profile parameters in early pregnancy in those women with and without stress incontinence on visual analogue scores (VAS) according to Cutner (1993). Median values, inter-quartile ranges and ranges are shown

In addition, the urethral pressure profilometry data revealed a correlation between the length of the first stage and deterioration in urethral parameters postnatally. We found that the maximum urethral closure pressure, maximum urethral pressure,

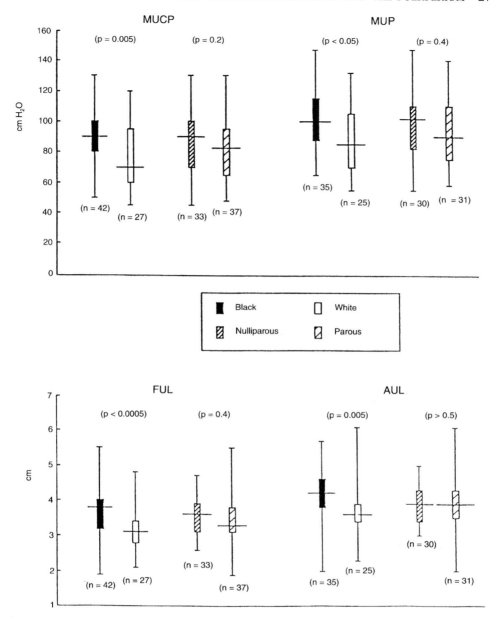

Figure 2.7   Urethral pressure profile parameters in early pregnancy according to race and parity (Cutner 1993). Median values, inter-quartile ranges and ranges are shown

functional urethral length and anatomical urethral length were significantly greater in black women compared to white women postnatally. This would support the argument that susceptibility antenatally results in postnatal manifestation of sphincter damage in those women with adverse delivery factors.

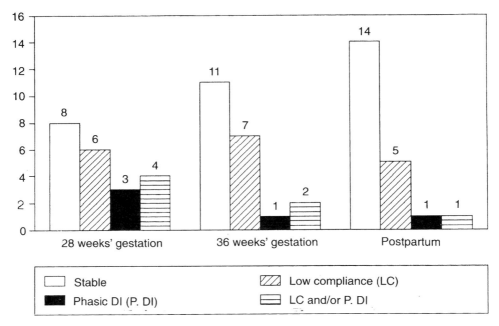

Figure 2.8   The number of women with detrusor instability (DI) on each occasion (Cutner 1993)

Until recently, only one author (Clow 1975) had performed subtracted provocative cystometry in pregnant women. He investigated 25 women, 15 of whom developed stress incontinence in pregnancy. Three of these had detrusor instability and the bladder became stable in these women in the puerperium.

Recently, we have demonstrated the occurrence of detrusor instability in pregnancy (Cutner 1993). We examined 75 women in early pregnancy and 23 (32%) had low compliance and 18 (24%) phasic detrusor instability. The women with low compliance had a significantly reduced first sensation and bladder capacity compared to women with a stable bladder and a significantly reduced bladder capacity compared to women with phasic detrusor instability (Table 2.3). In addition, those women with phasic detrusor instability had a significantly greater prevalence of urethral instability compared to low compliance and stable groups. These findings suggest that low compliance and phasic detrusor instability have a different aetiology in pregnancy, the former being an effect of uterine pressure and the latter due to inherent irritability. The cause of the latter may be related to high progesterone levels.

The prevalence of detrusor instability both during and after pregnancy from longitudinal data is shown in Figure 2.8. We found the prevalence antenatally to be significantly greater than that postpartum (Cutner 1993). It would thus appear that detrusor instability is an entity in pregnancy with improvement once the pregnancy is complete.

Thus it can be seen that stress incontinence is a common transient feature in pregnancy but most studies suggest that it resolves postpartum. The effects of pregnancy and mode of delivery on its genesis remain uncertain. From our own observations, race is an important factor which has not always been taken into account. Those studies which only examined the women postpartum are misleading as it may be the relative change which is of paramount importance, rather than exact values. Some studies cite urethral sphincter incompetence as the cause of stress incontinence in pregnancy, whilst our own work has demonstrated an increased prevalence of detrusor instability.

It would thus appear that stress incontinence in pregnancy and the postpartum period may be due to two different pathological processes, with detrusor instability as the cause during pregnancy, and genuine stress incontinence in the postpartum period.

Prevention and treatment

If antenatal stress incontinence is physiological and has no long-term sequelae, then reassurance is all that is required. However, this transient symptom may be a marker for possible long-term problems. It would now appear irrefutable that in susceptible women, a long protracted labour results in permanent genuine stress incontinence and if we were able to identify this group of women, an elective Caesarean section may be justified. To subject all women with antenatal stress incontinence to an abdominal delivery would lead to an unacceptably high Caesarean section rate as, in some cases, incontinence is due to detrusor instability and in others it will merely be transient.

When the equation of morbidity and mortality of elective Caesarean section versus an intended vaginal delivery is compared, one must also include the effects of an emergency Caesarean section and the later morbidity and mortality of an incontinence operation. If all parameters were included, then an elective Caesarean section in an 'at risk' group may be justified. At the present time there is one small group where elective Caesarean section should be advised. These are women who have undergone an effective incontinence procedure prior to pregnancy.

The present trend of 'natural labour' with long first stages and no time limit for the second stage may need to be questioned in the future if it is found that there is an unacceptably high prevalence of urethral sphincter damage. It is possible that a more liberal use of episiotomy and earlier recourse to forceps delivery would help to prevent some cases of sphincter damage. This is only speculation and further work is necessary before such a policy could be instituted.

A simple, non-invasive preventive measure may be the more formal teaching of pelvic floor exercises. However, if a muscle is already damaged, then pelvic floor training is unlikely to be effective.

Anticholinergic therapy for detrusor instability in pregnancy could not be justified and the rigours of bladder drill would be unacceptable to patients with a temporary condition. However, incontinence persisting postnatally should be investigated.

Voiding difficulties

Urinary retention in pregnancy is an uncommon event and usually due to an impacted retroverted uterus, classically occurring at 16 weeks' gestation. The cause is probably the result of the pelvic tumour (enlarged uterus) preventing the normal opening mechanisms of the internal urethral meatus. Treatment is catheterisation and then manual correction of the uterus into an anteverted position using a ring or Hodge pessary. Subsequently, voiding difficulties must be looked out for as over-distension may have resulted in detrusor damage and require long-term catheterisation until recovery occurs.

Symptoms of voiding difficulties appear to be fairly common in pregnancy (Figures 2.2, 2.3) but their cause is merely a function of small volumes of urine being passed (Cutner 1993). We found no difference in the peak flow rate or average flow rate between those women with and without the symptom of a slow stream or incomplete bladder emptying once the volume voided was taken into account.

Several studies have tried to determine the effects of delivery on both detrusor and urethral function. Weil *et al.* (1983) assessed 27 primigravid women urodynamically 2–5 days postpartum. They were divided into three groups: vaginal delivery without epidural analgesia, vaginal delivery with epidural analgesia, and lower segment Caesarean section. The Caesarean section group had a lower bladder capacity compared to the other two groups and the epidural group had a greater prevalence of hypotonic bladders and larger bladder capacities than either of the other two groups.

Recently, it has been demonstrated that after epidural analgesia, the bladder takes up to eight hours to regain its sensation and within this time period more than one litre of urine may be produced (Khullar and Cardozo 1993). This would result in detrusor damage.

Postpartum retention may result in long-term sequelae. Care of the bladder following delivery requires particular vigilance. Attention should be paid to those patients at risk of developing retention including those who have had a traumatic delivery, prolonged labour, epidural analgesia or Caesarean section. Voiding alone is not adequate assessment of bladder function since it may be incomplete, leading to increasingly large residuals of urine. Input–output charts are generally inadequate following delivery as a diuresis may occur and women are encouraged to increase their fluid intake to promote breastfeeding. Ideally, with an epidural, an in-dwelling catheter should be inserted and left in situ for 12 hours after the last top-up.

Thus, epidural analgesia, and traumatic vaginal delivery may lead to the development of acute urinary retention. Its sequelae of long-term voiding difficulties postpartum are preventable by a policy of early catheterisation if retention is suspected.

Summary

Lower urinary tract symptoms antenatally are almost universal and in most cases transient. The symptom of stress incontinence may be produced by physiological changes in the bladder neck support mechanism or due to detrusor instability. Retention of urine is one of the few conditions which must be treated in the antenatal period as there will be long-term sequelae. Women who have undergone a successful anti-incontinence procedure should have an elective Caesarean section. In labour, there should be liberal use of catheterisation to prevent long-term consequences. Most cases of incontinence are transient and investigation should be delayed until at least six weeks postpartum. However, if the patient complains of a continuous leak, then investigation is mandatory to exclude retention with overflow or urinary fistulae.

References

Allen, R.E., Hosker, G.L., Smith, A.R.B. and Warrell, D.W. (1990) Pelvic floor damage and childbirth: a neurophysiological study. *Br J Obstet Gynaecol* **97**, 770–9

Clow, W.M. (1975) Effect of posture on bladder and urethral function in normal pregnancy. *Urol Int* **30**, 9–15

Cutner, A. (1993) The lower urinary tract in pregnancy. MD Thesis. University of London

Dimpfl, Th., Hesse, U. and Schussler, B. (1992) Incidence and cause of postpartum urinary stress incontinence. *Eur J Obstet Gynecol Reprod Biol* **43**, 29–33

Francis, W.J.A. (1960) Disturbances of bladder function in relation to pregnancy. *J Obstet Gynaecol Br Empire* **67**, 353–66

Iosif, S., Ingemarsson, I. and Ulmsten, U. (1980) Urodynamic studies in normal pregnancy and in puerperium. *Am J Obstet Gynecol* **137**, 696–700

Iosif, S. and Ulmsten, U. (1981) Comparative urodynamic studies of continent and stress incontinent women in pregnancy and in the puerperium. *Am J Obstet Gynecol* **140**, 645–50

Khullar, V. and Cardozo, L.D. (1993) Bladder sensation after epidural analgesia. *Neurourol Urodyn* **12**, 424–5

Landon, C.R., Crofts, C.E., Smith, A.R.B. and Trowbridge, E.A. (1990) Mechanical properties of fascia during pregnancy: a possible factor in the development of stress incontinence of urine. *Contemp Rev Obstet Gynaecol* **2**, 40–6

Malpas, P., Jeffcoate, T.N.A. and Lister, U.M. (1949). The displacement of the bladder and urethra during labour. *J Obstet Gynaecol Br Empire* **56**, 949–60

Parboosingh, J. and Doig, A. (1973) Renal nyctohemeral excretory patterns of water and solutes in normal human pregnancy. *Am J Obstet Gynecol* **116**, 609–15

Stanton, S.L., Kerr-Wilson, R. and Harris, G.V. (1980). The incidence of urological symptoms in normal pregnancy. *Br J Obstet Gynaecol* **87**, 897–900

van Geelen, J.M., Lemmens, W.A.J.G., Eskes, T.K.A.B. and Martin, C.B. (1982) The urethral pressure profile in pregnancy and after delivery in healthy nulliparous women. *Am J Obstet Gynecol* **144**, 636–49

Weil, A., Reyes, H., Rottenberg, R.D. *et al.* (1983) Effect of lumbar epidural analgesia on lower urinary tract function in the immediate postpartum period. *Br J Obstet Gynaecol* **90**, 428–32

3

Female urinary incontinence –
which patients? – which tests?

Gerald J. Jarvis

Introduction

Female urinary incontinence is a common problem. In a recent community survey 14% of women questioned had been incontinent of urine at some time, the majority within the previous two months (Brocklehurst 1993). In one such incontinent population assessed urodynamically, 65% of patients had genuine stress incontinence, 18% detrusor instability, and 17% had both (Keane *et al.* 1992). In general, a diagnosis is made in clinical medicine by taking an accurate history and examining the patient. This process is then supplemented by appropriate investigation.

In deciding upon the cause of urinary incontinence in women, these principles apply less well than in many other areas of medicine. There are two major reasons for this. The first is the appreciation that the term 'stress incontinence' is a symptom and not a diagnosis. It is commonly associated with the condition of genuine stress incontinence but it is not pathognomonic of that condition. Similarly, the term 'urge incontinence' is a symptom and is commonly found in the condition of detrusor instability but again it is not pathognomonic of that condition. As shown in Table 3.1, when the symptoms are considered for 100 consecutive patients with genuine stress incontinence and 100 consecutive patients with detrusor instability, there is gross overlap between the symptoms complained of by patients with either condition (Jarvis 1990). Secondly, a patient may interpret different events by means of a common symptom. Thus, urgency is defined as a strong and sudden desire to void and this may be due either to an involuntary detrusor contraction, i.e. detrusor instability, or due to the sensation of urgency from bladder proprioceptors which may be associated with anxiety, infection or stone. This chapter will discuss the indications for urodynamic investigation in incontinent women and will then give guidance as to the place of different methods of urodynamic investigation.

Table 3.1 Symptoms and diagnosis

Symptoms	Genuine stress incontinence (n = 100)	Detrusor instability (n = 100)
Frequency	57	86
Nocturia	29	80
Urgency	46	92
Urge incontinence	37	98
Stress incontinence	99	26

Which patients?

There is now a wealth of evidence to demonstrate that clinical diagnosis, when assessed objectively by a urodynamic assessment, is accurate in approximately 70% of patients only. Glenning (1984) demonstrated that the cause of incontinence was only clinically correct in 56% of patients. Other workers have suggested a clinical diagnostic accuracy of 58% (Sand *et al.* 1988), 76% (Jarvis *et al.* 1980), 81% (Versi *et al.* 1991), and 87% (Lagro-Janssen *et al.* 1991). When the available published information is combined by means of meta-analysis, the overall diagnostic accuracy in genuine stress incontinence is only 69.2% whilst the overall diagnostic accuracy in detrusor instability is only 70.4%.

When those symptoms as shown in Table 3.1 are reassessed, it becomes clear that if a patient complains of stress incontinence and no other symptom, she approaches a 100% chance that the diagnosis is genuine stress incontinence and such a patient could be treated on the clinical diagnosis providing she has had no previous surgery. Similarly, if the patient complains of urgency and urge incontinence but no stress incontinence, she approaches a 100% chance that the diagnosis is detrusor instability providing that there are no stigmata of local urological or neurological disease.

However, such pure histories are relatively uncommon. In one series, only 12 out of 494 women with the symptom of stress incontinence had this as the sole symptom. In the other 482 patients, a urodynamic study was necessary in order to obtain an accurate diagnosis (Haylen *et al.* 1989). The problem arises in the vast majority of patients where the symptom of stress incontinence coexists with either urgency and/ or urge incontinence. If a patient complains of stress incontinence and urgency, however mild that urgency might be, she has a 90% chance of having detrusor instability and it seems unreasonable to treat such a patient surgically without a preliminary urodynamic assessment. Similarly, if the patient complains of the triad of stress incontinence, urgency and urge incontinence then she has a 60% chance of genuine stress incontinence and a 40% chance of detrusor instability, a situation in which it is clearly impossible to make a clinical diagnosis and a urodynamic assessment is mandatory (Jarvis 1990). Thus, we now have the first indication for a urodynamic assessment:

- all patients who complain of urgency prior to surgery for supposed genuine stress incontinence.

In those patients who did have a pure history, empirical therapy may have been commenced. No treatment in any form for urinary incontinence is successful in all patients and if treatment is not successful in the first instance, it would seem unreasonable to persist with further treatment unless the diagnosis had been confirmed urodynamically. It is well known that no operation for genuine stress incontinence will make 100% of patients continent whilst no drug or behavioural therapy for detrusor instability will also be universally effective. Treatment failure must always be considered as a potential indication for either initial urodynamic investigation or repeat urodynamic investigation.

This is particularly true should further surgery be contemplated, since it is well recognised that patients with detrusor instability have been operated on in the erroneous belief that they had genuine stress incontinence (Farrar *et al.* 1975). Moreover, every surgical procedure which has been described for genuine stress incontinence is associated with a demonstrable post-operative incidence of detrusor instability which had not been present pre-operatively. As a generalisation, the more obstructive an operation, the greater is the incidence of post-operative *de novo* detrusor instability such that it has been described in less than 1% of patients following a bladder buttress procedure (Beck *et al.* 1991), 6% of patients following a Stamey endoscopic bladder neck suspension (English and Fowler 1988), 10% following bladder sling (McGuire *et al.* 1987), and in 14% of patients following a colposuspension (Galloway *et al.* 1987). Only following a urodynamic assessment could the further management of such patients be planned scientifically.

Thus, we now have the second and third indications for urodynamic investigation:

- all patients who are thought to have an unstable bladder but are failing to respond to treatment;
- patients who are incontinent despite surgery for genuine stress incontinence.

There are three further indications for a urodynamic assessment, although perhaps less common in clinical gynaecological practice. The first relates to the possibility of voiding difficulties since the classical symptoms of hesitancy, poor stream, difficulty in voiding or incomplete emptying are only associated with objective voiding dysfunction in one third of such patients (Stanton *et al.* 1983). All patients who have urinary symptoms and a spinal injury should undergo both a urodynamic assessment and radiological or ultrasound imaging of the whole of the urinary tract, whilst patients who are to be included in a scientific series should ideally have undergone a urodynamic assessment before entry into a trial in order that the diagnosis is confirmed and a second assessment following treatment in order that results are objectively and not subjectively assessed.

Summary

Indications for urodynamics

1 When symptom of stress incontinence is accompanied by urgency of incontinence.
2 When medical treatment has failed.
3 When surgical treatment has failed.
4 When voiding dysfunction is suspected.
5 When a spinal injury is present.
6 When a scientific evaluation of treatment is being performed.

Which tests?

The range of urodynamic investigations which are available is wide and is listed in Table 3.2. A urodynamic investigation should involve the assessment of the function and dysfunction of the urinary tract by any appropriate method. These are dynamic investigations since continence and incontinence are dynamic processes. Static investigations, such as intravenous urography and cystoscopy, are not indicated unless there is an additional indication for their performance. Every patient does not require every test; a critical review of the indications for, and the limitation of, each test should allow the most appropriate selection to be made for each patient. Ideally, urodynamic investigations should be performed, or at a minimal level

Table 3.2 Urodynamic investigations

Pad weighing	Pressure-flow studies
Q-tip test	Urethral pressure profilometry
Filling cystometry	Urethral electrical conductance
Ambulatory urodynamics	Electromyography
Videocystourethrography (VCU)	Sacral nerve studies
Ultrasound	Bladder cooling test
Fluid bridge test	

supervised, by a clinician with a direct involvement in treating urinary incontinence. Only with such a system can the clinician who receives a report have sufficient confidence in it to allow it to be used as a basis for further clinical management.

The performance of each investigation requires standardisation in both technique and terminology if errors are to be avoided and information understood. These should conform to the recommendations of the International Continence Society (International Continence Society Committee on Standardisation of Terminology 1990).

The urodynamic examinations listed in Table 3.2 will now be discussed in this chapter and in the next chapter.

Pad weighing

This test is designed to quantify urine loss under standard and reproducible conditions. Having emptied her bladder, the patient wears a pre-weighed absorbent nappy or pad, drinks 500 ml of liquid over a 15-minute period, and then performs a series of tasks including walking, climbing stairs, coughing, and handwashing, over a 60-minute period. The pad is then re-weighed and the urine loss recorded in grams. Sometimes the diuresis is delayed and the test results should then be expressed at both 60 and 120 minutes. Should voluntary voiding occur, it should be measured and recorded separately.

This test will confirm that the patient is, in fact, incontinent and may give a guide as to the severity of that involuntary urine loss (Sutherst *et al.* 1981). Not all patients who complain of urinary incontinence are in fact incontinent during either a cystometric or a videocystourethrographic examination but if incontinence can be demonstrated using a pad test then the examination should be repeated. This may occur in up to 6% of patients (Jorgensen *et al.* 1987). Most investigators believe that there is a good correlation between the weight of fluid on the pad and the severity of incontinence as described by the patient (Sutherst *et al.* 1986; Victor *et al.* 1987) although a minority of authors would disagree with this view (Kinn and Larsson 1987). Some clinicians believe that the style of the incontinence as described by the patient gives a guide to the diagnosis, patients with detrusor instability leaking larger volumes of urine but at less frequent intervals than do patients with genuine stress incontinence. The pad test has shown that there is very little evidence to support this clinical impression (Sutherst *et al.* 1986).

The main indications for a pad test, therefore, are to quantify urine loss either before or after treatment, or to confirm incontinence on a patient who is not incontinent during a more formal urodynamic investigation.

Q-tip test

This test has never achieved any degree of popularity in the UK but has some popularity in North America where it is considered to be an 'office procedure'.

The principle of this test is that a cotton-tipped swab is placed into the urethra such that its tip is at the urethrovesical junction. The patient is asked to strain and the angle of the arc made by the distal end of the Q-tip is measured. The larger the arc, the greater is the mobility of the bladder neck and the assumption is made that the cause of the patient's incontinence is genuine stress incontinence (Crystle *et al.* 1972). However, more serious investigation has failed to demonstrate any correlation between the degree of mobility and the differential diagnosis between genuine stress incontinence and detrusor instability (Fantl *et al.* 1986; Karram and Bhatia 1988).

This test would seem to contribute nothing to that already available from clinical examination.

Filling cystometry

Filling cystometry is probably the single most useful investigation in deciding whether the patient has genuine stress incontinence or detrusor instability, or both. It is the method by which the pressure–volume relationship of the bladder is measured, assessing detrusor activity, sensation, capacity and compliance. The underlying principle is that the pressure exerted by the detrusor is measured during the filling phase. The detrusor pressure cannot be measured. The total pressure within the bladder is the sum of the abdominal pressure and the detrusor pressure. Both the abdominal pressure (measured with a rectal sensor) and the total bladder pressure (measured with an intravesical sensor) can be measured and displayed continuously whilst electronic subtraction will result in a continuous real-time read-out of detrusor pressure. In general, the bladder is filled with sterile saline or radio-opaque medium via a urethral catheter at up to 100 ml per minute. Both bladder pressure and abdominal pressure are measured continuously using either fluid-filled lines or microtransducers inserted via the urethra and rectum. The patient should assume a standing position at some stage during the test and provocations designed to elicit positive changes (e.g. coughing, heel-rolling) should occur (Bates *et al.* 1970).

The detrusor pressure should not alter appreciably during filling. Any rise in pressure, especially one which mimics the patient's symptoms, should be recorded along with the first desire to micturate (generally 100–200 ml) as should the maximum cystometric capacity (generally over 450 ml). If urine leakage is noted in the presence of raised intra-abdominal pressure but in the absence of detrusor activity, genuine stress incontinence may be diagnosed. If the detrusor pressure rises and falls in a phasic manner either spontaneously or on provocation whilst the patient is trying to inhibit micturition, detrusor instability is diagnosed. Sometimes the detrusor pressure rises continuously rather than in a phasic manner. Such a finding is termed reduced compliance and is treated as a variant of detrusor instability. It is taken for granted that the patient is awake, unanaesthetised, and not taking any drugs which affect bladder function.

There are some important features concerning the conduct and interpretation of a filling cystometrogram. The test itself is reproducible if saline or radio-opaque medium is used (Ramsden *et al.* 1977). There was a vogue for the use of carbon dioxide as a filling medium in that it was less messy but partly due to the inability to diagnose leaks in the system and partly due to the effect of the gas upon the lower urinary tract itself, large variations in quantitative cystometric data became apparent and a failure to generate reproducible data has resulted in an abandonment of this filling medium (Wein *et al.* 1978). Not every patient who complains of urinary incontinence will have an abnormality demonstrated by filling cystometry. In general, this is due to a failure to demonstrate detrusor instability. The technique of provocation cystometry is now in common practice in order to stimulate involuntary detrusor contractions and hence demonstrate detrusor instability. Such provocation includes filling at up to 100 ml per minute and alterations in the posture of the patient during filling. Although provocation is not physiological, it does seem to enable the test to generate the information which is required since a stable detrusor cannot be provoked to contract. Without such provocation, detrusor instability will be missed in up to 50% of patients with this condition (Awad and McGuinnis 1983; Jarvis 1981; Ramsden *et al.* 1977). In the interests of economy, some units have attempted to use single channel cystometry (recording the total bladder pressure only) in the belief that this could be interpreted in order to distinguish between genuine stress incontinence and detrusor instability. Should there be genuine stress incontinence alone, then such a system may be used but should there be genuine stress incontinence and detrusor instability, detrusor instability alone, or a patient who is straining perhaps to avoid urinary leakage during the procedure, then an erroneous result may be used for patient management (Ouslander *et al.* 1988).

In summary, any investigative regime used to assess a patient with urinary incontinence will include a filling cystometrogram.

Ambulatory urodynamics

There is good evidence to show that abnormalities can be demonstrated in a subgroup of patients, in whom no abnormality is demonstrable on normal studies. Some 90% of patients in whom no diagnosis was available following a filling cystometrogram will have a diagnosis following an ambulatory cystometrogram. It may be anticipated that those abnormalities will include detrusor instability alone (57%), genuine stress incontinence alone (30%), or both coexisting (13%) (McInerney *et al.* 1991; van Waalwijk *et al.* 1991; Webb *et al.* 1991).

Ambulatory urodynamics is covered in more detail in the following chapter.

Videocystourethrography (VCU)

In this test, a filling cystometrogram is performed with radiological screening of the bladder and urethra using an image intensifier (Bates *et al.* 1970). Although the combined test is no better than a filling cystometrogram alone in distinguishing between genuine stress incontinence and detrusor instability, it has the advantages of easier visualisation of leakage, the assessment of the position and mobility of the bladder neck (especially after previous surgery), the estimation of residual urine, and an opportunity to diagnose morphological abnormalities such as bladder or urethral diverticulae, urethral stenosis, or vesico-ureteric reflux which may be present in up to 7% of incontinent patients (Benness *et al.* 1989; Shepherd 1990).

In current practice, therefore, VCUs could be safely reserved for more complicated cases such as patients in whom previous surgery has failed, patients in whom routine urodynamic investigations have given equivocal results and ambulatory urodynamics is not available, or in patients with neurological dysfunction. The disadvantages of VCUs include the expense and sophistication of the equipment, the assistance of a radiographer and radiologist which may result in less versatility in running a clinical service, and the potential risk of irradiation to the patient whilst the staff wear radiation protection. By recording these studies on videotape, they are particularly useful for teaching purposes.

Ultrasound

The use of ultrasound in order to observe the bladder neck during a filling cystometrogram avoids the potential risk of irradiation and reduces the cost of equipment. It is simpler and quicker than a VCU and perhaps is better accepted by the patients.

Initially, the use of a transvaginal probe was advocated in order to observe the opening and descent of the bladder neck (Quinn *et al.* 1988) but it is possible that the physical presence of an ultrasound probe within the vagina may distort the variables being investigated. There is evidence that the use of a vaginal probe may compress and stretch the urethra with an artificial elevation of the bladder neck at rest, an inability to judge the full degree of descent of the bladder neck during straining, and the distortion of some urethral pressure profile variables including an apparent increase in maximum urethral closure pressure, functional urethral length, and an increase in the area under a pressure profile (Wise *et al.* 1992). However, these disadvantages may be overcome by the use of transrectal ultrasound which does not induce artefacts (Richmond and Sutherst 1989; Yamada *et al.* 1991).

A more important criticism of this technique is that if ultrasound is the only investigation used in patients with urinary incontinence, genuine stress incontinence may be seen by immediate bladder neck opening on straining whereas detrusor instability is only implied by this study and may allow erroneous judgements to be made. This may be overcome by combining ultrasound imaging of the bladder neck with a filling cystometrogram (Koelbl and Bernaschek 1989).

The point of combining some form of imaging techniques with a filling cystometrogram and not relying on the imaging technique alone is a very valid one. There is now good evidence that even apparently normal continent women have an incompetent bladder neck but maintain continence by use of their distal urethral sphincter. An open bladder neck at rest has been reported in up to 24% of nulliparous asymptomatic women and in up to 50% of continent women during straining (Chapple *et al.* 1989; Versi 1991; Versi *et al.* 1986). It is therefore mandatory that genuine stress incontinence or detrusor instability are not simply diagnosed because urine leaks from the bladder into the proximal urethra. The urine leakage must reach beyond the distal sphincter mechanism or else incontinence cannot be said to occur and otherwise apparently normal women will undergo unnecessary treatment.

Fluid bridge test

This test was designed to identify the presence of urine in the proximal urethra in the presence of a cough and an incompetent sphincter mechanism. When this occurs, fluid forms a bridge between the pressure and the proximal urethra and hence if pressures are measured at both those positions they will be identical at that moment. The test was designed to diagnose genuine stress incontinence in the absence of fluid leaking along the whole of the urethral length and out of the external urethral meatus (Sutherst and Brown 1980). However, it has already been stated that an incompetent bladder neck is not the same as genuine stress incontinence and hence there will be a significant false-positive rate from this procedure (28%) representing the incidence of an incompetent proximal sphincter mechanism in the absence of genuine stress incontinence in the population under study. This test has not found widespread use.

Pressure-flow studies

These studies assess the dynamics of urine flow, generally measured by recording detrusor pressure during voiding and the maximal urine flow rate (in millilitres per second) and the time during which flow occurred by asking the patient to void into a collecting vessel with a metal strip capacitor. As a generalisation, the volume voided should also be measured since the voiding variables are inconsistent if the volume is below 200 ml. Obstructed voiding is characterised by a high detrusor pressure achieving a low flow rate but the combination of a low detrusor pressure with a low flow rate indicates a hypotonic detrusor which may be due to numerous different factors including neurological damage and long-standing untreated obstruction.

As a generalisation, women void at a higher flow rate than men but exert a lower detrusor pressure. A normal study might be characterised by detrusor pressures below 40 cm of water associated with a flow in excess of 20 ml per second. There is also a fall in maximum flow rate as age increases.

The major value of uroflowmetry lies in the prediction of post-operative voiding difficulties in patients with genuine stress incontinence. Up to 22% of women with genuine stress incontinence have an asymptomatic coexisting voiding disorder and this is associated with difficulty in voiding following surgery together with a longer duration of catheterisation (Bergman and Bhatia 1985; Haylen et al. 1990). At a minimum level, the clinician who has identified an asymptomatic voiding disorder prior to surgery for genuine stress incontinence may forewarn the patient of some delay in achieving satisfactory voiding post-operatively and at a more serious level may wish to avoid a surgical procedure associated with a high incidence of obstruction in such patients. Sadly, there is a close correlation between the percentage of patients made continent by a given operative procedure and the incidence of post-operative voiding difficulty, perhaps because many operations work, to some degree, by creating an outlet obstruction. A bladder buttress is rarely if ever associated with long-term voiding problems whereas they occur in approximately 5% of patients following a Stamey endoscopic bladder neck suspension (Vordermark et al. 1979), 10% of patients following a bladder sling (Enzelsberger et al. 1990), and in up to 23% of patients following a colposuspension (Lose et al. 1987).

It could therefore be argued that all patients who are to undergo surgery for genuine stress incontinence should have a urodynamic voiding study performed pre-operatively in order to influence the choice of operative procedure offered.

Urodynamic studies in clinical practice

The most commonly used tests are filling and voiding cystometry. Filling cystometry is generally able to distinguish between genuine stress incontinence and detrusor instability or identify when both are present. Urine flow rates are able to screen for asymptomatic disorders. Imaging of the lower urinary tract gives additional information on morphology but is not necessarily essential to clinical practice. The other investigations described above are useful in specific circumstances but not in all patients.

The history is really only a guide to the severity of the symptoms whereas a urodynamic investigation is diagnostic. Shepherd (1990) reported that when the referring consultant acted upon the recommendation of the urodynamic assessment, 72% of the patients were cured or significantly improved whereas when the treatment was at variance with that recommended by the urodynamic assessment, only 38% were cured or improved.

A urodynamic assessment is, however, time-consuming, potentially unpleasant for the patient, expensive, and carries an appreciable morbidity. Some 5% of women find the investigation distasteful and some series have reported post-urodynamic dysuria in 48% of patients, frequency in 39%, haematuria in 37%, and bacteriologically-proven urinary tract infection in 19% (Baker *et al.* 1991; Coptcoat *et al.* 1988). The use of prophylactic antibiotics (such as nitrofurantoin 50 mg four times a day for one day or trimethoprim 200 mg once) will reduce the incidence of bacteriologically-proven urinary tract infection by 66% (Baker *et al.* 1991; Coptcoat *et al.* 1988).

Conclusion

There are specific indications for urodynamic investigations and these have been discussed above together with the place of each investigation. It is not possible to escape from the conclusion that urodynamic investigations are acceptable to the majority of patients and will improve both diagnostic accuracy and clinical outcome.

References

Awad, S.A. and McGuinnis, R.H. (1983) Factors that influence the incidence of detrusor instability in women. *J Urol* **130**, 114–15

Baker, K.R., Drutz, H. and Barnes, M.D. (1991) Effectiveness of antibiotic prophylaxis in prevention of bacteriuria after multi channel urodynamics. *Am J Obstet Gynecol* **165**, 679–81

Bates, C.P., Whiteside, C.G. and Turner-Warwick, R.T. (1970) Synchronous cine/pressure/flow/cystourethrography with special reference to stress and urge incontinence. *Br J Urol* **42**, 714–23

Beck, R.P., McCormick, S. and Nordstrom, L. (1991) 25-year experience with 519 anterior colporrhaphy procedures. *Obstet Gynecol* **78**, 1011–18

Benness, C.J., Barnick, D.J. and Cardozo, L.D. (1989) Is there a place for routine videocystourethrography in the assessment of lower urinary tract dysfunction? *Neurosurgery and Urodynamics* **8**, 299–300

Bergman, A. and Bhatia, N.N. (1985) Uroflowmetry for predicting post-operative voiding difficulties in women with genuine stress incontinence. *Br J Obstet Gynaecol* **92**, 835–8

Brocklehurst, J.C. (1993) Urinary incontinence in the community. *BMJ* **306**, 832–4

Chapple, C.R., Helm, C.W., Blease, S. *et al.* (1989) Asymptomatic bladder neck incompetence in nulliparous females. *Br J Urol* **64**, 357–9

Coptcoat, M.J., Reed, C., Cumming, J. *et al.* (1988) Is antibiotic prophylaxis necessary for routine urodynamic investigations? *Br J Urol* **61**, 302–3

Chrystle, D., Charm, L. and Copeland, W. (1972) Q-tip test in stress urinary incontinence. *Obstet Gynecol* **38**, 313–15

English, P.J. and Fowler, J.W. (1988) Videourodynamic assessment of the Stamey procedure for stress incontinence. *Br J Urol* **62**, 550–2

Enzelsberger, H., Schatten, C., Kurz, C. and Fitzal, P. (1990) Urodynamic and radiologic parameters before and after loop surgery for recurrent urinary stress incontinence. *Acta Obstet Gynaecol Scand*, **69**, 51–4

Fantl, J.A., Hurt, W.G., Bump, R.C. *et al.* (1986) Urethral axis and sphincter function. *Am J Obstet Gynecol* **155**, 554–8

Galloway, N.T.M., Davis, N. and Stephenson, T.P. (1987) The complications of colposuspension. *Br J Urol* **60**, 122–4

Glenning, A.B. (1984) Clinical symptoms and urodynamic assessment. *Aust N Z J Obstet Gynaecol* **24**, 95–7

Haylen, B.T., Sutherst, J.R. and Frazer, M.I. (1989) Is the investigation of most stress incontinence really necessary? *Br J Urol* **64**, 147–9

Haylen, B.T., Parys, B.T., Anyaebunam, W.F. *et al.* (1990) Urine flow rates in male and female urodynamic patients compared with the Liverpool normogram. *Br J Urol* **65**, 483–7

International Continence Society Committee on Standardisation of Terminology (1990) The standardisation of terminology of lower urinary tract function. *Br J Obstet Gynaecol* **97**, Suppl. 6, 1–16

Jarvis, G.J. (1981) Urodynamics. *Lancet* **i**, 497

Jarvis, G.J. (1990) 'The place of urodynamic investigation' in G.J. Jarvis (Ed.) *Female Urinary Incontinence*, pp. 15–20. London: Royal College of Obstetricians and Gynaecologists

Jarvis, G.J., Hall, S., Stamp, S. *et al.* (1980) An assessment of urodynamic examination in continent women. *Br J Obstet Gynaecol* **87**, 893–6

Jorgensen, L., Lose, G. and Andersen, J.T. (1987) One hour pad weighing test for objective assessment of female urinary incontinence. *Obstet Gynecol* **69**, 39–42

Karram, M.M. and Bhatia, N.N. (1988) The Q-tip test. *Obstet Gynecol* **71**, 807–11.

Keane, D.P., Eckford, S.D., Shepherd, A.M. and Abrams, P. (1992) Referral patterns and diagnoses in women attending a urodynamic unit. *BMJ* **305**, 1438

Kinn, A.C. and Larsson, B. (1987) Pad test with fixed bladder volume and urinary stress incontinence. *Acta Obstet Gynaecol Scand* **66**, 369–71

Koelbl, H. and Bernashek, G. (1989) A new method for sonographic urethrocystography and simultaneous pressure flow measurements. *Obstet Gynecol* **74**, 417–22

Lagro-Janssen, A.L.M., Debruyne, F.M.J. and Van Weel, C. (1991) Value of the patient's case history in diagnosing urinary incontinence in general practice. *Br J Urol* **67**, 569–72

Lose, G., Jorgennsen, L., Mortensen, S.O., Molsted-Petersen, L. and Krisense, J.K. (1987) Voiding difficulties after colposuspension. *Obstet Gynecol* **69**, 33–8

McGuire, E.J., Bennett, C.J., Konnak, J.A., Sonda, P.A. and Savastano, J.A. (1987) Experience with pubovaginal slings for urinary incontinence at the University of Michigan. *J Urol* **138**, 525–6

McInerney, P.D., Vanner, T.F., Harris, S.A.B. and Stephenson, T.P. (1991) Ambulatory urodynamics. *Br J Urol* 272–4

Ouslander, J., Leach, G., Abelson, S. *et al.* (1988) Simple versus multi channel cystometry in the evaluation of bladder function in an incontinent geriatric population. *J Urol* **140**, 1482–6

Quinn, M.J., Benyon, J., Mortensen, N.J.M. and Smith, P.J.B. (1988) Vaginal endosonography in the post-operative assessment of colposuspension. *Br J Urol* **63**, 295–300

Ramsden, P.D., Smith, J.C., Pierce, J.M. and Ardran, G.M. (1977) The unstable bladder – fact or artefact? *Br J Urol* **49**, 633–9

Richmond, D.H. and Sutherst, J.R. (1989) Transrectal ultrasound scanning in urinary incontinence. *Br J Urol* **64**, 582–5

Sand, P., Hill, R.C. and Ostergard, D.R. (1988) Incontinence history as a predictor of detrusor instability. *Obstet Gynecol* **71**, 257–60

Shepherd, A. (1990) 'The range of urodynamic investigation' in G.J. Jarvis (Ed.) *Female Urinary Incontinence*, pp. 21–31. London: Royal College of Obstetricians and Gynaecologists

Stanton, S.L., Ozsoy, C. and Hilton, P. (1983) Voiding difficulty in the female: prevalence, clinical and urodynamic review. *Obstet Gynecol* **61**, 144–7

Sutherst, J.R. and Brown, M.C. (1980) Detection of urethral incompetence in women using the fluid bridge test. *Br J Urol* **52**, 138–42

Sutherst, J.R., Brown, M.C. and Shawer, M. (1981) Assessing the severity of urinary incontinence in women by weighing perineal pads. *Lancet* **i**, 1128–30

Sutherst, J.R., Brown, M.C. and Richmond, E. (1986) Analysis of the pattern of urine loss in women with incontinence as measured by weighing perineal pads. *Br J Urol* **58**, 273–8

van Waalwijk, E.S.C., Remmers, A. and Janknegl, R.A. (1991) Extramural ambulatory urodynamic monitoring during natural filling and normal daily activities. *J Urol* **146**, 123–41

Versi, E. (1991) The significance of an open bladder neck in women. *Br J Urol* **68**, 42–3

Versi, E., Cardozo, L.D., Studd, J.W.W. *et al.* (1986) Internal urinary sphincter maintenance of female continence. *BMJ* **292**, 166–7

Versi, E., Cardozo, L., Anand, D. and Cooper, D. (1991) Symptom analysis for the diagnosis of genuine stress incontinence. *Br J Obstet Gynaecol* **98**, 815–19

Victor, A., Larrson, G. and Asbrink, A.S. (1987) A simple patient administered test for objective quantification of the symptom of urinary incontinence. *Scand J Urol Nephrol* **21**, 277–9

Vordermark, J.S., Brannen, G.E., Wettlaufer, J.N. and Modarelli, R.O. (1979) Suprapubic endoscopic vesical neck suspension. *J Urol* **122**, 165–7

Webb, R.J., Ramsden, P.D. and Neal, D.E. (1991) Ambulatory monitoring and electronic measurement of leakage in the diagnosis of detrusor instability. *Br J Urol* **68**, 148–52

Wein, A.J., Hanno, P.M., Dixon, D.O. *et al.* (1978) The reproducibility and interpretation of carbon dioxide cystometry. *J Urol* **120**, 205–6

Wise, B.G., Burton, G., Cutner, A. *et al.* (1992) Effects of vaginal ultrasound probe on lower urinary tract function. *Br J Urol* **70**, 12–16

Yamada, T., Mizuu, T., Kawakami, S. *et al.* (1991) Application of transrectal ultrasound in modified Stamey procedure for stress urinary incontinence. *J Urol* **146**, 1555–8

4

Complex investigations in urodynamics

David M. Holmes

One of the pitfalls of clinical investigation is our tendency to measure a physiological function purely because we have the technology to do so, rather than considering how the measurement will affect our management decisions. It is in our patients' best interest to minimise the number of investigations we carry out to those which are strictly necessary in order to decide on a course of management.

A Test is the recording of measurements of a physiological function. These measurements are compared with normal values, and the result indicates what course of action should be taken, i.e. the results of the test allow a decision to be made.

An Investigation is also a measurement of a physiological function, but the information which it gives, though no doubt interesting, is not itself relevant to the decision-making process.

The tests which have been defined in urogynaecology are as follows:

1 Completing a urinary diary, which allows us to make the diagnosis of urinary frequency.
2 A pad test, which allows us to make the diagnosis of incontinence.
3 Filling cystometry, which allows us to make the diagnosis of either genuine stress incontinence or detrusor instability.

The methodology for carrying out these tests has been clearly defined and their diagnostic criteria are well described.

Many other 'complex' investigations have been described, among them the following:

Lateral bead chain cystogram
Retrograde sphincterometry
Urethral pressure (fluid perfusion and microtip)
Urethral sensitivity
'Q'-tip test
Urethral strain gauge
Pressure fluid bridge
Electric fluid bridge
Urethral electric conductance (DUEC and BNEC)
Electromyography
Ultrasound
MRI/CT scanning
Ambulatory monitoring

Urethral pressure, conductivity studies and ambulatory monitoring have been selected for discussion: urethral pressure, because it is an investigation already incorporated into clinical practice; conductivity, because the author was fortunate to be involved with some of the early work in this area and ambulatory monitoring because this seems to be the way forward.

The lateral bead chain cystogram was first described by Hodgkinson, the 'father' of modern urodynamics, in 1958 (Hodgkinson *et al.* 1958). Over 30 years on from this he produced a fairly damning indictment of subsequent urethro-vesical function investigations. In 1990 he said that, 'Many techniques had been introduced, none are specific and few are standardised' (Hodgkinson 1990). Whenever an investigation of urethro-vesical function is performed his words should be kept in mind.

It is well recognised that the bladder has two purposes. It functions as a reservoir for the storage of urine but also has the complementary function of expulsion of urine. The vast majority of investigations are guided towards the investigation of the failure of its storage function, i.e. urinary incontinence.

Urinary leakage can only occur if:

1 the detrusor muscle contracts involuntarily
2 there is involuntary urethral relaxation, or
3 there is a failure of transmission of intra-abdominal pressure to the urethra.

It is important to realise that urinary leakage can occur by any combination of these factors, and that the diagnosis of genuine stress incontinence and detrusor instability can be made during the same cystometry.

Cystometry measures the detrusor pressure, but does not measure what is happening in the urethra when leakage occurs. The diagnosis of genuine stress incontinence is made by failing to observe detrusor activity rather than by positively identifying inefficient abdominal pressure transmission.

Measurement of urethral pressure

The measurement of urethral pressure would seem to be a complementary investigation to cystometry. Bonney referred to retrograde sphincterometry as far back as 1923 (Bonney 1923), but it was not until 1967 that Toews first described the fluid perfusion technique of measuring pressure in the urethra (Toews 1967). Her technique was an adaptation of the fluid perfusion technique previously used to measure oesophageal pressure and which was subsequently modified by Brown and Wickham in 1969 (Brown and Wickham 1969) and remains in clinical use. Fluid perfusion involves the use of a side hole catheter through which a fluid is forced at a constant rate. The pressure required to lift the urethral wall away from the side hole of the catheter and maintain this constant flow is measured and can be displayed.

A more convenient method for estimating urethral pressure is a microtip pressure transducer. The miniaturised pressure sensor measures the accumulation of forces on the transducer face. Two transducers may be combined on one catheter, allowing the simultaneous measurement of both intravesical and intra-urethral pressures. The disadvantage of the fluid perfusion methods of measuring urethral pressure is their low frequency response which precludes measurement of fast events such as a cough. The catheters can, however, be made very flexible, thus reducing the well-described

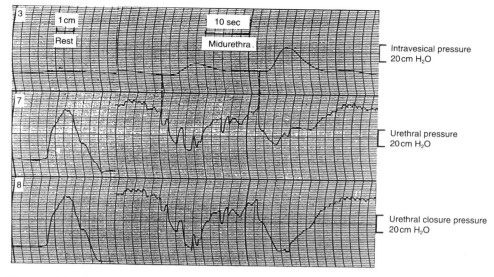

Figure 4.1   Resting urethral pressure profile (left) and continuous urethrocystometry (right) in a patient with idiopathic detrusor instability (courtesy of Mr Paul Hilton)

artifacts due to the inherent stiffness of the microtip transducers. Microtip transducers have a high-frequency response and therefore can measure cough transmission and it is for this reason that they have gained in popularity. They are also much more 'user friendly' than the fluid perfusion techniques.

The three possible investigations of urethral pressure are:

1 to measure the pressure at a single point in the urethra over a period of time;
2 to measure the pressure throughout the length of the urethra whilst it is quiescent;
3 to measure the pressure in the urethra throughout its length whilst estimating how much intra-abdominal pressure is transmitted to the urethra at various points along its length.

Single point measurement of urethral pressure

Here the transducer is held at the point of maximum pressure and the variations of pressure recorded over a period of time. Variations in urethral pressure are found in women with both detrusor instability and sensory urgency (Kulseng-Hanssen 1983; Plevnik and Janez 1983) and so cannot be used to distinguish between detrusor instability and a stable bladder. The example illustrated in Figure 4.1 shows pressure measured in mid-urethra with a fixed volume of fluid in the bladder of a woman who has unstable detrusor contractions. There are large variations in pressure over the course of time. Note that the urethral pressure falls just prior to an unstable contraction. The finding of a drop in urethral pressure occurring in the absence of a detrusor contraction has led to the description of 'urethral instability', the clinical significance of which is uncertain.

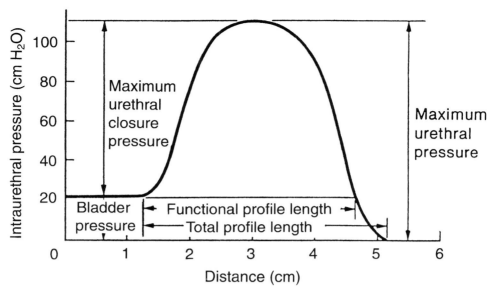

Figure 4.2   A schematic representation of the urethral closure pressure profile (ICS 1988)

Static urethral pressure profile

The second method of investigating urethral pressure is to pull the transducer through the urethra at a fixed speed whilst measuring the pressures in both the bladder and the urethra. This generates a profile of urethral pressure along the urethra. The International Continence Society has defined the landmarks on the profile shown in Figure 4.2 (Abrams *et al.* 1988). The functional profile length is the length of the urethra where the urethral pressure exceeds intravesical pressure and urethral closure pressure is the difference between bladder pressure and urethral pressure at any point along the profile.

   The profile illustrated in Figure 4.3 was obtained by Toews in 1967. The International Continence Society landmarks are clearly demonstrated. It is interesting to note that even at this stage an attempt was made to obtain a stress profile. This is a normal pressure profile. Toews also took three groups of women: those who had no symptoms of stress incontinence; those who had mild stress incontinence, and those who had severe stress incontinence. She plotted their urethral pressure profiles and calculated the mean profiles for each group. These are illustrated in Figure 4.4. It can be seen that the maximum urethral closure pressure increases clearly with decreasing symptoms. It is also apparent that there is no correlation between the severity of symptoms and the functional urethral lengths. Hilton standardised the technique of urethral pressure measurement using microtip transducers and in 1981 produced a very similar graph, shown in Figure 4.5 (Hilton and Stanton 1983). Urethral pressure is plotted against urethral length in two

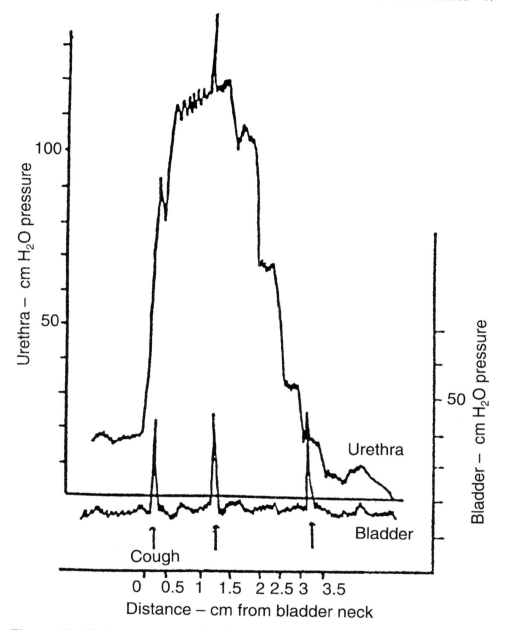

Figure 4.3   Resting pressure profile of bladder and urethra of normal subject (Toews 1967)

groups of women: those who were symptom free and those who had genuine stress incontinence. The profiles are plotted ± two standard deviations. The overlap is so large that it is not possible confidently to distinguish the urethral pressure profile of an incontinent woman from that of a continent woman.

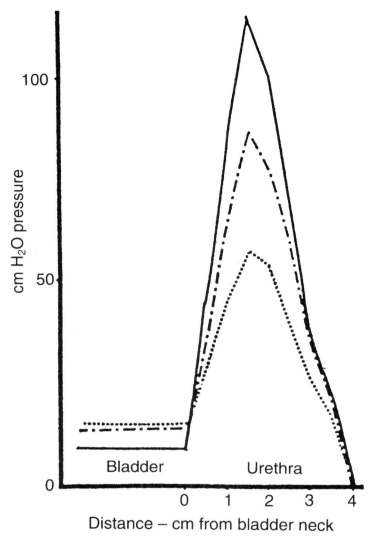

Figure 4.4 Mean resting pressure and urethral pressures in normal subjects and in stress incontinent patients. Solid line indicates normal; dashed line, mild stress incontinence; dotted line severe stress incontinence (Toews 1967)

Stress urethral pressure profile

The stress urethral pressure profile relies on the fact that urine will only leak if intravesical pressure exceeds intra-urethral pressure. Intravesical pressure is equal to the sum of the detrusor pressure and intra-abdominal pressure, whilst intra-urethral pressure is the sum of the intrinsic pressure exerted by the urethral sphincter mechanism plus whatever percentage of the intra-abdominal pressure is transmitted to the urethra at that point. An efficient transmission will give a value of 100%, whilst inefficient transmission gives rise to a lower value. The first example shown

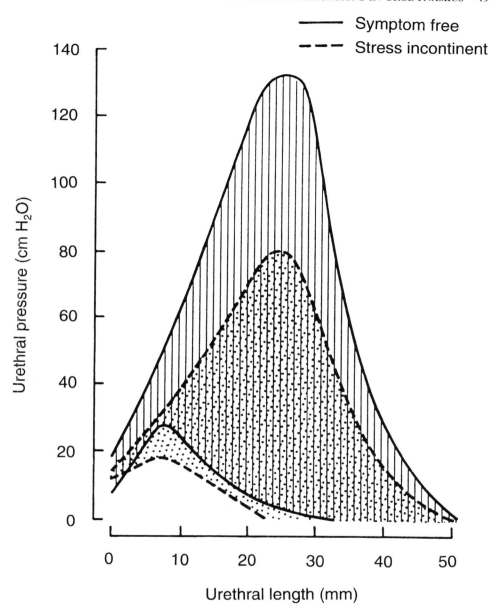

Figure 4.5 Resting urethral closure pressure profiles in stress incontinent and symptom free women. Profiles are constructed from mean ± 2 standard deviations for conventional profile parameters (Hilton 1983)

in Figure 4.6 is of a symptom-free woman. The left-hand side shows the static urethral pressure profile with its characteristic shape. The central profile is obtained by withdrawing the catheter at a fixed speed whilst the woman coughs every few seconds. The coughs are clearly seen on the intravesical pressure and urethral pressure tracings. The equipment also calculates the urethral closure pressure by subtracting

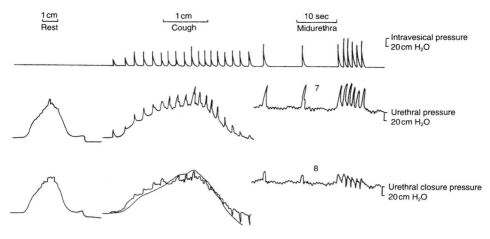

Figure 4.6   Resting and cough profiles in symptom free woman (courtesy of Mr Paul Hilton)

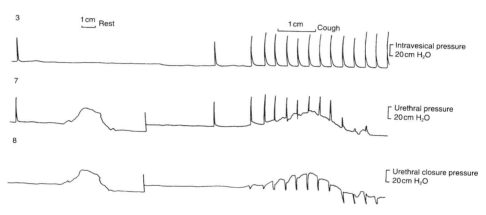

Figure 4.7   Resting and cough profiles in woman with genuine stress incontinence (courtesy of Mr Paul Hilton)

intravesical pressure from urethral pressure. A negative deflection on the urethral closure pressure suggests that there is an inefficiency in pressure transmission at that point. A positive deflection suggests that there has been augmentation of pressure transmission. There is much debate as to the nature of this augmentation. It would seem that it is either a result of reflex contraction of the fast twitch fibres of the rhabdo-sphincter, or a reproducible artefact due to catheter stiffness. The right-hand tracings are obtained from leaving the pressure transducer at mid-urethra and gauging the response to coughing. The next tracing (Figure 4.7) shows a woman who has genuine stress incontinence. Again the left-hand trace shows a static urethral pressure profile, whilst the right-hand tracing shows the dynamic or stress profile. Note the consistent negative deflections on the urethral closure pressure which infer failure of pressure transmission. A negative value of the closure pressure infers that stress incontinence would occur. Versi (1990) has performed sophisticated statistical analysis of virtually every measurement of urethral pressure of 172 women. Unfortunately, no clear distinction can be made between those women who have genuine stress incontinence and those who have a competent sphincter mechanism. The best measure for separating the presence and absence of genuine stress incontinence is discriminant analysis of all the measurements, but the overlap persists, thus precluding clinical use of urethral pressure profilometry to identify genuine stress incontinence.

Why should we continue to measure urethral pressure?

There is no doubt that urethral pressure measurement is a useful research tool which can give us a good idea of the methods of action of intervention in the management of genuine stress incontinence. It must, however, be seen as an investigation rather than a test of urethral function, and at present should probably not influence clinical decision making.

It has been recognised that a low maximum urethral closure pressure correlates with a poor surgical outcome. This was first reported by McGuire in 1981 and other authors since then (McGuire 1981; Sand *et al.* 1987). More recently a number of authors have suggested that the value of the maximum urethral closure pressure at a static profile indicates which sort of surgery should be used to cure the abnormality (Blaivas and Olsson 1988; Bowen *et al.* 1989; Koonings *et al.* 1990). The inference is that finding a maximum urethral closure pressure of less than 20 cm of water is an indication for carrying out a sling procedure (Horbach *et al.* 1988). The validity of this hypothesis is yet to be properly tested, but if it is proven, then there may be a reason to perform pressure profiles.

If urethral pressure cannot replace cystometry, why do we need to pursue other tests further? One of the problems with cystometry is its poor correlation with symptoms. Abrams (1983) noted that 70% of people with normal cystometry complained of urgency, whilst Cardozo (1984) noted that 55% of women with genuine stress incontinence complained of stress and urge incontinence whilst 35% of women with detrusor instability also had mixed symptoms. It has also been reported that 10% of asymptomatic women have evidence of detrusor instability (Turner-Warwick 1979), though no large series of cystometries on normal women has been published. This has given rise to Jarvis's much quoted statement of the bladder being 'an unreliable witness' (Jarvis *et al.* 1980). What must also be asked is whether cystometry is an unreliable test?

Urethral electrical conductance (UEC)

Plevnik first described impedance measurements in the lower urinary tract in 1981 (Plevnik and Vrtacnik 1981). In 1985 the original device was redesigned and consists of two gold-plated ring electrodes mounted on a fine silastic catheter (Plevnik *et al.* 1985). A 20 millivolt peak-to-peak, 50 kHz signal is generated across these electrodes and the resulting current which flows is measured. The extent of the field is 6.5 mm

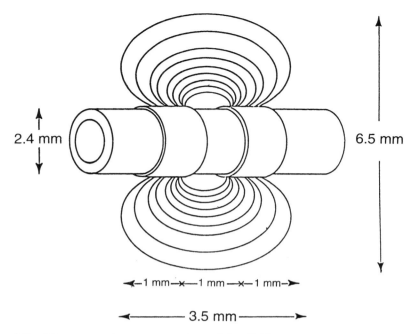

Figure 4.8   Diagrammatic representation of the field around the UEC electrodes in saline

from side to side when the electrodes are in saline (Figure 4.8). If anything of a low impedance impinges, the current will fall proportionally. The catheter fixation device is fixed on the short catheter and is movable on the long catheter. If the electrodes are placed in a saline-filled bladder and slowly drawn through the bladder neck mechanism through the external urethral orifice, then a profile of urethral electrical conductance or, more strictly, impedance is generated. The current which flows when the electrodes are bathed in saline is high and rapidly falls as the electrodes come through the relatively low impedance area of the urethra. A superimposed static urethral pressure profile is illustrated in Figure 4.9. Note that the first fall of urethral electrical conductance occurs before there is a rise in the urethral pressure. The inference is that this area is the bladder neck mechanism. If the electrodes are left at the bladder neck mechanism whilst monitoring detrusor pressure in a woman who has spontaneous involuntary detrusor contractions it is seen that there is much activity at the bladder neck mechanism (Figure 4.10). The woman has been asked to indicate those times at which she feels an increase in the sensation of urgency and these are marked on the chart. Every time she had an unstable contraction she marks an increase in the sensation of urgency. She also marks times when there is no increase in detrusor pressure and these coincide with increases in conductivity, inferring that the bladder neck has opened at this point. There has been no detrusor pressure rise to account for this.

This phenomenon was used in a test which would give a measurement correlating better with the symptom of urgency than conventional cystometry (Holmes *et al.* 1989). A group of 23 consecutive women with varying symptoms of stress and urge incontinence had their symptoms graded. The maximum detrusor pressure rise found

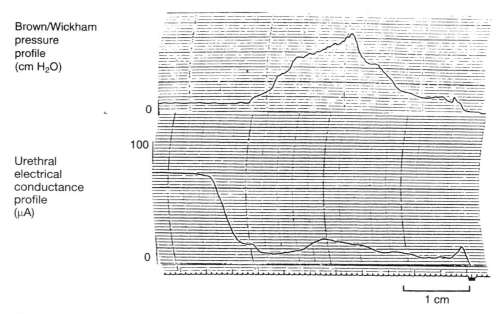

100

Brown/Wickham
pressure
profile
(cm H$_2$O)

0

100

Urethral
electrical
conductance
profile
(μA)

0

1 cm

Figure 4.9 Superimposition of simultaneously derived UEC and Brown–Wickham profiles (Holmes 1989)

during cystometry was recorded. The new test consisted of the women lying in the dorsal position with 250 ml of saline in the bladder. The electrodes of a UEC catheter were left at the bladder neck mechanism and the maximum deflection from peak to trough over a time period of one minute was measured. This was used as the test measurement. Increasing urgency against the maximum detrusor pressure rise is illustrated in Figure 11(a). Note that a significant number of women who have severe symptoms of urgency have normal detrusor pressure rises, whilst some women who have no urgency were found to have detrusor instability. When the new test data were correlated with increasing symptoms of urgency, as shown in Figure 4.11(b), it is seen that there is a highly significant correlation between increasing symptoms and increasing activity at the bladder neck mechanism. A cut-off of 13 microAmps distinguishes those who have urgency.

Bringing the electrodes more distal in the urethra and fixing them at 1.5 cm from the external urethral orifice allows measurement of leakage below the point of maximum urethral pressure. They are held in position by the catheter fixation device whilst the woman is asked to cough and exercise. Leakage has been successfully identified by this method (Creighton *et al.* 1991). Three different patterns of leakage have been identified and are postulated to represent different aetiologies of leakage. Peattie *et al.* (1988) added a DUEC catheter whilst measuring detrusor pressure at a maximum cystometric capacity during conventional cystometry in 104 women. They showed a good correlation between the patterns of leakage and the cystometric diagnosis. Illustrated in Figure 4.12 are tracings showing: (a) a type 1 pattern and

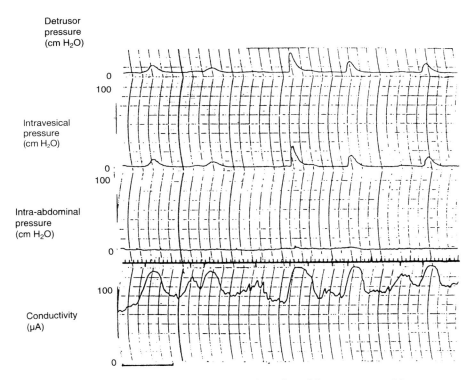

Figure 4.10   Bladder neck conductivity variations found in a woman with spontaneous, idiopathic detrusor instability (Holmes 1989)

genuine stress incontinence; (b) a type 3 pattern demonstrating detrusor instability; and (c) a combination of types 1 and 3 demonstrating both DI and GSI. The fourth trace (d) suggests a diagnosis of urethral instability, and indeed this may be the case.

Should DUEC replace cystometry?

Every new test has its protagonists and antagonists. Peattie and colleagues (1988) believe that DUEC performed '... simultaneously with cystometry should be part of the standard urodynamic work-up ...'.

Mayne and Hilton (1987) felt that these patterns of leakage were not diagnostic and merely represented the volume of fluid loss. Clearly, the opinion is split as to whether the DUEC is a worthwhile investigation and more research in this area is needed.

Intra-operative use of the UEC catheter

A novel use of the UEC catheter was described by Janez and Plevnik (1989). They used the UEC catheter intra-operatively to determine how tight to make the sutures when carrying out a Stamey procedure. Epidural anaesthesia is required and once

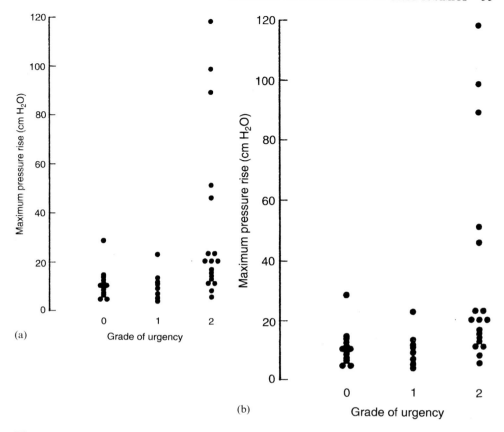

Figure 4.11 Correlation between subjective symptoms of urgency and (a) maximum detrusor pressure rise during cystometry; (b) maximum deflection of conductivity at rest (Holmes 1989)

the sutures are in place the UEC probe is held at the bladder neck. The sutures are slowly tightened whilst the patient is coughing until such time as the bladder neck is seen to close. This allows minimal tension on the sutures and hopefully will reduce the recognised failure rate of the procedure.

Ambulatory monitoring

The technique of continuous monitoring of detrusor function introduced by James (1979) increases the detection rate of involuntary contractions in symptomatic women who have normal cystometry (James 1984; McInerney *et al.* 1990). This appears to change their diagnostic category to that of detrusor instability. In 1983 James used this technique on 320 incontinent women; 43% had incontinence due to involuntary detrusor function (James 1983). He found an increase in the rate of detection of unstable contractions from 36.5% quoted for the investigation of 800 women by conventional cystometry (Cardozo 1984), thus indicating an increased sensitivity.

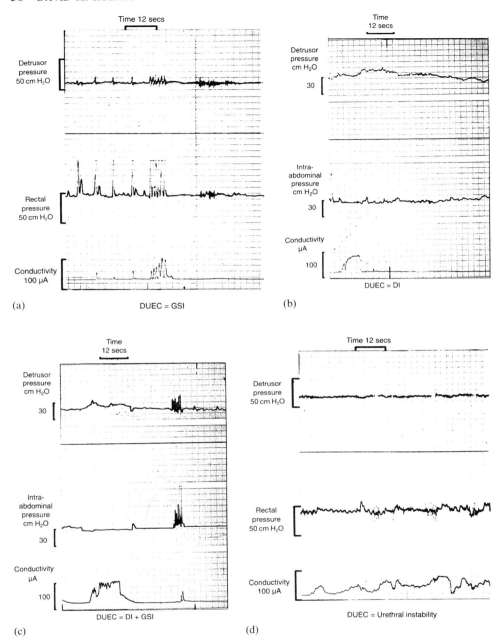

Figure 4.12   DUEC at maximum cystometric capacity with the cystometric diagnosis of: (a) genuine stress incontinence; (b) detrusor instability; (c) genuine stress incontinence and detrusor instability; (d) presumed urethral instability (courtesy of Dr Alison Peattie)

Only three women appeared to leak without evidence of intravesical pressure rises. The aetiology of their incontinence is presumed to be urethral instability (Ulmsten *et al.* 1977). Similar increased rates of motor urge incontinence of 42.2% have been reported (van Waalwijk van Doorn *et al.* 1987).

The upsurge in interest in ambulatory monitoring has been brought about by the introduction of the micro-processor systems, which allow computer analysis of detrusor and urethral function (Janknegt *et al.* 1989; Bailey *et al.* 1989; Mulder and Vierhout 1991). These systems have been used to try to define what 'normal' detrusor function is under these circumstances. Thirty female and three male asymptomatic volunteers have been assessed over a mean of 5.52 hours (Robertson *et al.* 1991). Of these only 36% had completely stable detrusor function. Thirty per cent exhibited five or more unstable contractions, mostly appearing just before micturition. These findings have been substantiated by other investigators. Clearly, this technique will give us much information about 'normal' bladder function but great caution should be exercised in applying the same diagnostic criteria used in cystometry to the results of ambulatory monitoring.

Urinary incontinence is a benign condition and so our patient's symptoms are of paramount importance. The ideal test would detect abnormalities which are associated with those symptoms, but as yet no test of urethro-vesical function is perfect. In this situation we should use investigations to back up our clinical diagnosis rather than to replace it.

References

Abrams, P., Blaivas, J.G., Stanton, S.L. and Andersen, J. (1988) The standardisation of lower urinary tract function. *Scand J Urol Nephrol (suppl)* **114**, 5–19

Abrams, P.H. (1983) 'The clinical contribution of urodynamics', in P.H. Abrams, R.C.L. Fenley and M. Torrens (Eds) *Urodynamics*, p. 142. London and Berlin: Springer-Verlag

Bailey, R., Abrams, P., Shepherd, A.M. and Bailey, D. (1989) Development of a micro-computer based system for long term ambulatory monitoring using data-reduction. *Neurourol Urodynamics* **8**, 403

Blaivas, J. and Olsson, C.A. (1988) Stress incontinence: classification and surgical approach. *J Urol* **139**, 727–31

Bonney, V. (1923) On diurnal incontinence of urine in women. *J Obstet Gynaecol Br Empire* **30**, 358–65

Bowen, L.W., Sand, P.K. and Ostergard, D.R. (1989) Unsuccessful Burch retropubic urethropexy: a case controlled urodynamic study. *Am J Obstet Gynecol* **160**, 452–8

Brown, M. and Wickham, J.E.A. (1969) The urethral pressure profile. *Br J Urol* **41**, 211–17

Cardozo, L.D. (1984) 'Detrusor instability', in S.L. Stanton (Ed.) *Clinical Gynecologic Urology*, pp. 193–203. St Louis: Mosby

Creighton, S.M., Plevnik, S. and Stanton, S.L. (1991) Distal urethral electrical conductance (DUEC) – a preliminary assessment of its role as a quick screening test for incontinent women. *Br J Obstet Gynaecol* **98**, 69–72

Hilton, P. and Stanton, S.L. (1983) Urethral pressure measurement by micro-transducer: the results in symptom-free women and in those with genuine stress incontinence. *Br J Obstet Gynaecol* **90**, 919–33

Hodgkinson, C.P., Doub, H. and Keely, W. (1958) Urethro-cystograms: metallic bead technique. *Clin Obstet Gynecol* **1**, 668–77

Hodgkinson, C.P. (1990) The renaissance of female urethrovesical function. *Int Urogynecol J* **1**, 104–8

Holmes, D.M., Plevnik, S. and Stanton, S.L. (1989) Bladder neck electrical conductivity in female urinary urgency and urge incontinence. *Br J Obstet Gynaecol* **96**, 816–20

Horbach, N.S., Blanco, J.S., Ostergard, D.R. *et al.* (1988) A suburethral sling procedure with polytetrafluoroethylene for the treatment of genuine stress incontinence in patients with low urethral closure pressure. *Obstet Gynecol* **71**, 648–752

James, E.D. (1979) Continuous monitoring. *Urol Clin North Am* **6**, 125–35

James, E.D. (1983) The bladder during physical activity: further views on natural-filling urodynamic investigations. *Br J Urol* **55**, 570

James, E.D. (1984) 'Ambulatory monitoring in urodynamics', in A.R. Mundy, T.P. Stephenson and A.J. Wein (Eds) *Urodynamics – Principles, Practice and Application*, pp. 120–6. Edinburgh: Churchill-Livingstone

Janez, J. and Plevnik, S. (1989) Urethral electric conductance (UEC) controlled Stamey procedure. *Neurourol Urodynamics* **8**, 338–9

Janknegt, R.A. and van Waalwijk van Doorn, E.S.C. (1989) Clinical experiences with advanced ambulatory urodynamics. *Neurourol Urodynamics* **8**, 402–4

Jarvis, G.J., Hall, S., Stamp, S. *et al.* (1980) An assessment of urodynamic examination in incontinent women. *Br J Obstet Gynaecol* **87**, 893–6

Koonings, P.P., Bergman, A. and Ballard, C.A. (1990) Low urethral pressure and stress urinary incontinence in women: risk factor for failed retropubic surgical procedure. *Urol* **36**, 245–8

Kulseng-Hanssen, S. (1983) Prevalence and pattern of unstable urethral pressure in 174 gynecologic patients referred for urodynamic investigation. *Am J Obstet Gynecol* **146**, 895–900

Mayne, C.J. and Hilton, P. (1987) A comparison of distal urethral electrical conductance (D.U.E.C.) with weighed pads during a standardised exercise test. *Neurourol Urodynamics* **6**, 167–8

McGuire, E.J. (1981) Urodynamics findings in patients after failure of stress incontinent operations. *Prog Clin Biol Res* **78**, 351–60

McInerney, P.D., Vanner, T.F., Powell, C.S. and Stephenson, T.P. (1990) Ambulatory urodynamics. *Neurourol Urodynamics* **9**, 381–2

Mulder, A.F.P. and Vierhout, M.E. (1991) Combined ambulatory urodynamics and pad testing. *Neurourol Urodynamics* **10**, 420–2

Peattie, A.B., Plevnik, S. and Stanton, S.L. (1988) Distal urethral electric conductance (DUEC) test: a screening test for female urinary incontinence? *Neurourol Urodynamics* **7**, 173–4

Plevnik, S. and Vrtacnik, P. (1981) Electric fluid bridge test. *Proc 11th Meeting Int Continence Soc*, Lund, pp. 56–7.

Plevnik, S. and Janez, J. (1983) Urethral pressure variations. *Urol* **21**, 207–9

Plevnik, S., Holmes, D.M., Janez, J. *et al.* (1985) Urethral electric conductance (UEC) – A new parameter for the evaluation of urethral and bladder function: methodology of the assessment of its clinical potential. *Proc 15th Meeting Int Continence Soc*, London, pp. 90–1

Robertson, A.S., Griffiths, C.J., Ramsden, P.D. and Neal, D.E. (1991) Ambulatory monitoring and conventional urodynamic studies in normal volunteers. *Neurourol Urodynamics* **10**, 418–19

Sand, P.K., Bowen, L.W., Panganiban, R. and Ostergard, D.R. (1987) The low pressure urethra as a factor in failed retropubic urethropexy. *Obstet Gynecol* **69**, 399–402

Toews, H. (1967) Intra-urethral and intravesical pressures in normal and stress incontinent women. *Obstet Gynecol* **29**, 613–24

Turner-Warwick, R. (1979) Observations on the functions and dysfunctions of sphincter and detrusor mechanism. *Urol Clin North Am* **6**, 13–30

Ulmsten, U., Andersson, K-E. and Persson, C.G.A. (1977) Diagnostic and therapeutic aspects of urge urinary incontinence in women. *Urol Int* **32**, 88–96

van Waalwijk van Doorn, E.S.C., Zwiers, W., Wetzels, L.L.R.H. and Debruyne, F.M.J. (1987) A comparative study between standard and ambulatory urodynamics. *Neurourol Urodynamics* **6**, 159–60

Versi, E. (1990) Discriminant analysis of urethral pressure profilometry data for the diagnosis of genuine stress incontinence. *Br J Obstet Gynaecol* **97**, 251–9

5

The role of the urodynamics nurse

Jill Lord

Introduction

This chapter aims to illustrate that nurses in urodynamic units are capable of performing a much wider role than is the case in many units at the present time, and that this is beneficial to the patients, nursing staff and the medical staff.

Before discussing the role of the urodynamics nurse I would like to give you a brief description of the unit in which I work. The unit consists of a consultant, a principal physicist, a clinical nurse specialist, three staff nurses, two research registrars and secretarial staff. In addition to the urodynamic clinics there are a number of other clinics (see Table 5.1).

In total we see about 3500 patients each year, about 1500 of whom undergo urodynamic studies. The patients referred to the unit come from the whole of the North West region including Cumbria. They are referred to the unit by consultant gynaecologists, gynaecology outpatient departments, general practitioners and various sources including neurologists, urologists and geriatricians.

The role of the nurse

The role of the nurse within the unit can be described under the following headings:

Organisation of the unit
Urodynamics assessments
Nurse specialist clinics
Education and training
Research
Interdisciplinary communication

Table 5.1   Urological department activities

Urodynamic clinics
Ano-rectal physiology and EMG clinics
Cystoscopy clinics
Nurse specialist clinics
Maximal electrical stimulation clinic
Consultant clinics
Research registrar's clinics
Hysteroscopy clinics

Organisation of the unit

The clinics must be well organised as there are eight different types of clinic of which three may be running concurrently. This involves ensuring that the right resources are available for each clinic.

The 3500 patients seen annually are virtually all by prior appointment; this is approximately 15 patients for every working day.

Urodynamics assessments

One of the main functions of the nurse is performing urodynamic investigations on up to 30 patients per week. During these investigations there are no doctors present, the nurses do the history taking, investigations and interpretation of the results.

History taking

The interview is important to encourage the patient to give the information which can help to determine the correct diagnosis and management, in the time allocated. In taking the history we gather as much information about the patient and her symptoms as possible, to ensure that the most accurate diagnosis can be made.

It is important to have quiet and peaceful surroundings in which the patient feels comfortable and not threatened. It is often easier for female patients to talk to another female about their problem.

I try to be informal and friendly with patients, encouraging them to use my first name rather than 'Sister' and with the patient's permission I use her first name. I try to get the patient into a relaxed frame of mind, as she may well be anxious about her 'taboo' problem possibly because of unsympathetic attitudes displayed by society, relatives and even some members of the profession.

Although it is well known that many women have a urinary continence problem it is not normally discussed, even with relatives and close friends. They may feel uncomfortable going to their GP or any other medical practitioner, and may well have been suffering their problem for a considerable time before they come to a urodynamics department.

Many patients come with the attitude that no one can help with their problem, because previous experience has left them with that impression. During the introduction I try to assess the patient and what terminology she will understand, i.e. medical or layman's. This means finding out as much as possible about the patient in the limited time available.

I sit informally with the patient and explain that I am going to take a history and carry out the urodynamics tests, reassuring the patient that the procedures will be explained as the tests are conducted. One of the fears to be overcome is that of leaking during the tests. This explanation ensures that the patient realises that we understand her problem and the subsequent urodynamics tests proceed smoothly with the full co-operation of the patient leading to more accurate results. To keep the patient's confidence the same nurse who took the history will also introduce the catheters during the investigation.

To ensure sufficient time is given to each patient for the interview, we allow one hour – half an hour for the history taking and half an hour for the urodynamic

Table 5.2   Role of the nurse carrying out urodynamics

Uroflow
Cystometry
Urethrometry
Provocation
Voiding studies

tests, without interruption from telephones or colleagues. I take the history using a standard questionnaire, but I listen to the answers, adapting the next questions to what the previous answers may have revealed. The way that questions are asked is important, as is the use of language familiar to the patient. As most patients are not familiar with medical terminology of the lower urinary tract, we must use terms that are meaningful to them. Accuracy when recording answers is also important; for example, most patients when asked, will say that they are wet, but when questioned in detail it may be that they are only damp. It is important to record clearly and accurately the details of the interview as it may help later when evaluating the results of the tests, and for reference by the doctor who was not present during the history taking and will be reporting the results.

Carrying out urodynamics

Table 5.2 shows the order in which we usually perform the urodynamics tests, although this may be changed if we feel it is appropriate following on from the history taking. As we carry out the tests any slight abnormality is marked, and from our experience of performing many tests every week we are able to detect abnormalities which others may consider insignificant. For example:

(a)   It can be difficult to detect the difference between a urethral spasm and a stenosis when introducing catheters. A stenosis may indicate the need for urethral dilatation.

(b)   Similarly, on filling the bladder it is important to recognise if the patient has a urethral, bladder or suprapubic desire to void, as this could help to distinguish a urethral problem from a bladder problem.

(c)   A slight rise in detrusor pressure, which is easy to miss, can be important and it is therefore essential to detect and mark such rises. Such very slight rises can be an indication of bladder instability.

(d)   Observing the condition of urethral tissue can also provide valuable information, e.g. atrophy.

Recognising all such 'clues' and combining them with information gathered from the history taking helps to make a more accurate diagnosis.

Interpretation of results

The nursing staff are in part responsible for the interpretation of the results and communicating them to the doctor. In order to fulfil this role a detailed knowledge of the lower urinary tract is obviously essential. This knowledge must be obtained from a combination of formal courses, practical experience particularly working with the consultant and physicist, and reading technical journals and textbooks.

We use the International Continence Society terminology and the test results are compared with past, well-established data to check whether the patient's lower urinary tract activity is outside the normal values.

Nurse specialist clinics

The third function of the nurse is to hold nurse specialist clinics for the management of patients who in many units would be seen regularly by a clinician; here the nursing staff take on the complete management of the patient with selected reference to the consultant. This group of patients includes those who have built up a rapport with the named nurse and are comfortable and happy being managed, knowing that the nurse has the back-up of the consultant when necessary.

All patients attending the unit are encouraged to have telephone access to their named nurse should they have any problems or worries. This is part of our philosophy of gaining patient confidence, and the facility is extensively used by our patients.

The multiple sclerosis patient, for example, is advised on how to manage lower urinary tract dysfunction, including the use of catheters and medication to suit her life style. This is often done initially on an in-patient basis. For example, a young girl of 19 years with multiple sclerosis who has an active social life, requires to do intermittent self catheterisation and take oxybutinin tablets and use desmospray. I have advised her to take her oxybutinin 30 minutes prior to going out, and to do intermittent self catheterisation immediately before going out. This gives her four hours of being dry so that she is able to enjoy herself.

Another example is a young mother, 26 years old, also with multiple sclerosis who has three young children and can manage her incontinence when at home, but has difficulty when going shopping. I have advised her to take the oxybutinin tablets 30 minutes before she goes out. This will give her an adequate period of being dry to go out with her children without being worried about the location of the nearest toilet.

Another group of patients managed by the nurse specialist are women undergoing bladder retraining. Patients who require bladder retraining come into hospital for two weeks and are seen daily by the named nurse from the unit. They then return to the clinic for follow-up after two weeks, three months, six months and a year and are always reviewed by the same nurse. After this they are reviewed by the consultant and discharged.

For patients with chronic urinary problems we provide as much help as possible to improve and maintain their quality of life by providing management, advice and information on any relevant aids. The GPs of patients attending this clinic are kept informed of the progress and of any actions taken or required to help the patient.

Education and training

Another function of the nurse in the unit is education and training of health-care professionals and patients and carers.

Training of health-care professionals

We teach urodynamics to all health-care professionals including ward nurses, district nurses, continence advisers, specialist nurses and physiotherapists, all levels of medical staff and anyone else who may become involved with urodynamics.

We teach bladder management, including the fundamentals of lower urinary tract care, intermittent self catheterisation, and changing of suprapubic catheters. We provide an advisory service on the appropriate catheters, pads and other continence aids to use, taking into account the cost of these products. We provide information on the use of medication and aids, e.g. vaginal cones and vaginal sponges for the lower urinary tract. We advise community nurses on how to set up self-referral clinics, and how to conduct such clinics.

Training of patients

We advise patients about basic bladder management and health care, use of medication and aids as for the health-care professionals. We advise them about self care, including hygiene and do's and don'ts, for example, not to drink caffeine products.

We teach patients and carers the procedure of intermittent self catheterisation, how to change suprapubic catheters, to manage long-term in-dwelling urethral catheters and how to perform bladder washouts and the solutions to use.

Research

Another role of the nurse is to work closely with the medical staff and principal physicist in carrying out research into a wide range of topics connected with the function of the lower urinary tract, and the way urodynamics are carried out at other units in the UK (see below).

Examples of topics include the use of Reagent Stix for screening for urinary infection and provocative factors in the detection of detrusor instability.

Interdisciplinary communication

The urodynamics nurse can be used effectively as the focal point for interdisciplinary communication. To provide the best management for a patient it is important that all involved liaise to ensure that a full picture of individual problems is available when needed. Many problems fail to be addressed because one or other of the multidisciplinary team fails to communicate information to others. Sometimes important information is not passed on because of a failure to realise its importance. Failure to communicate information can lead to the patient's management being less effective than otherwise would be the case, so we try to ensure that the communication is effective.

Urodynamic personnel and training in the UK

As a unit at St Mary's Hospital in Manchester we were interested in evaluating how other units were operating and using their resources. We carried out a survey to determine the professional background of personnel carrying out urodynamics in the UK and whether they felt that they were adequately trained.

Of 171 questionnaires sent out, currently 94 have been returned. Two questions in the survey relate to the role of the nurse; 'Who takes the history?' and 'Who does the urodynamics investigations?' The results are shown below.

Who takes the history?

91% of all tests are preceded by taking a history.
77% of histories are taken by medical staff.
17% of histories are taken by nursing staff.
6% of histories are taken by others (technicians, physiotherapist, etc.).

Who does the urodynamics tests?

43% are done by doctors alone.
26% are done by doctors with nurses.
12% are done by nurses alone.
19% are done by others (technicians, radiographers, etc.).

I believe that this shows that the specialised skills and experience of nurses are underused. To fulfil this role nurses need extensive knowledge of the lower urinary tract. The nurse must also be a good listener and problem solver, and must have counselling skills.

Conclusion

In this chapter I have tried to show that nurses are capable of carrying out the urodynamics, including taking patient history and interpreting the test results. They are also able to hold specialist clinics for the management of patients.

This leads to benefits within the unit by giving the medical staff more time to devote to the things that only they can do, and thus the unit can deal efficiently with an increased number of patients.

The patients are satisfied because they have good quality of care, they always see the same member of staff and have more time devoted to them individually.

The nursing staff get more satisfaction through enhanced responsibility for urodynamics, running their own independent clinics, their teaching role, and the wider contact with other disciplines.

Our survey shows that only a small number of units are using nursing staff in the way that our unit does and many units are therefore not making the best use of their resources.

6

Cost and purchaser/provider considerations

Graham James

The purpose of this chapter is to look at the purchaser and provider issues in considering contracting for services, and in particular how new services or service developments are launched within the National Health Service since the 1991 NHS reforms.

Prior to 1991, district health authorities were allocated funds by their regional health authority, based on a series of calculations which quantified, in cash terms, the funding required to meet the health needs of the district's resident population. In turn, the district health authority would set budgets with each of the departments within its hospitals, community services or support services, for a 12-month period and the name of the game was to do as much activity as possible, without overspending the budget. Very few departments had budgets which related directly to activity and whether activity was greater or less than the previous year had no effect on the cash value of the budget. In other words, there was no penalty or incentive attached to the budget for productivity.

In respect of developing new services, or enhancing services already available, the clinical department would have three choices to secure the change:

1 Finance the development/change from within its own budget.
2 Bid to the senior officers of the health authority for the funding required to undertake the development/change.
3 Via their senior officers at the health authority, make a bid to the regional health authority for the funding to undertake the development/change.

As departmental budgets became tighter following the imposition of cost improvement programmes etc., the bidding process grew and this has had the effect of eradicating 'strategic' planning by a department or hospital, in favour of a 'stop–go' approach to service development dependent upon the focus the Department of Health or the regional health authority gives to a particular service in any particular year.

The internal market – 1991 NHS reforms

The reforms in 1991 changed this 'hit and miss' bidding system, by introducing an 'internal market' with purchasers and providers, the purchasers being district health authorities, regional health authorities in some instances for regionally purchased specialty services and GP fundholders. The focus of the reforms, was that purchasing

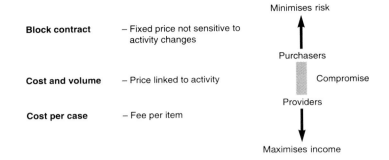

Figure 6.1   Purchaser and provider contracting perspectives

health authorities or GP fundholders, would set a purchasing plan into a contract which it would agree with a provider or providers, for a period of between 12 months and three years. This contracting process between purchasers and providers has, for the first time, created a formal link between activity and funding.

There are three basic forms of contracts that are currently utilised in the National Health Service, and these are:

1 **A block contract** – a contract which has indicative activity across a whole range of services and a fixed price which equates to the indicative activity. Should actual activity be higher or lower than the contract indicative volume, the price of the contract *does not* change. In other words, the contract is not volume sensitive.
2 **Cost and volume contract** – this type of contract creates a direct relationship between activity and price, usually again across a wide range of services. Where actual activity is greater than the volumes stipulated in the contract, then the purchaser would make additional payments to the provider over and above the contract price already being paid. Should activity fall below the contracted levels, then the provider would have to reimburse the purchaser a proportion of the contract price.
3 **Cost per case contract** – as the title suggests, this is a contract drawn up on a fee per item basis, in that, for each patient treated an individual charge is made by the provider to the purchaser. This type of contract is usually used for smaller contracts or single specialty arrangements and for patients who are treated outside a contractual arrangement at all (Extra Contractual Referrals). Most GP fundholder contracts would also fall into this category.

Contracting perspectives

The different perspectives that purchasers and providers would look at in trying to negotiate a contract to suit their needs, are shown in Figure 6.1.

Purchasers, in the main, will always prefer to minimise financial risk to themselves, as the resources made available to them are finite or cash limited. For this reason, purchasers will try and negotiate an arrangement similar to a block contract where the price is fixed irrespective of the level of activity undertaken by the provider.

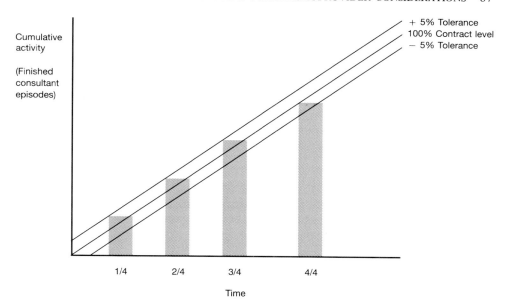

Figure 6.2 A contracted activity shown as 100% with 5% tolerance levels either side

Under this arrangement, the provider is at risk should they do more activity than is indicated in the contract, as they would not be paid, even at marginal costs, for this activity, whereas the purchaser has some risk because less than the indicative activity in a contract could be provided by a hospital, which would mean they had not received value for money for the amount paid.

The provider, on the other hand, will always want a close relationship between activity and contract price as, quite naturally, they want to be paid for each and every treatment they undertake. However, the administrative burden on managing cost per case contracts for a full range of services is so onerous that a compromise between the two is usually negotiated in the form of a cost and volume contract with tolerance levels at either side of the stipulated contracted activity. The tolerance levels are merely parameters within which the contract price would not change. Figure 6.2, for example, shows contracted activity as 100% with 5% tolerances at either side. If actual activity was at 95% of the contracted level, then the price would remain the same as it would if the contract was actually at 105% of the contracted level. Once activity falls below 95% or above 105%, then reimbursements or additional payments would be made accordingly.

The contracting perspectives of purchasers and providers can, therefore, be summarised as follows:

The purchaser wants the maximum service level at a good quality with minimal risk attached to the contract price.

The provider requires a tight relationship between price and activity for services at the highest affordable quality standards.

Service development/change

With this new contracting background, how does innovation and service development get launched?

It has to be said that the reforms have not made service development innovation and change easy. The provider must be able to negotiate additional income to cover the costs of development or change and, therefore, must be operating within a contracting environment that allows for a price change, i.e. not within a block contract arrangement. The purchaser, on the other hand, will want convincing of the patient benefits of the development or change, and will also require the implementation to offer value for money. Guidance from the NHS Management Executive suggests that the provider should develop a statement of case or 'business case' for presentation to potential purchasers who, at the end of the day, will make a decision as to whether or not to finance the development or change. A good business case will concentrate on six key issues:

1 Stating the clear patient benefits that will accrue due to the implementation of the development or change supported by good research data if possible.
2 A 'market analysis' i.e. data that show the district of residence of the estimated patient through-put as this will indicate which district health authorities or GP fundholders will need to be approached in order to finance the development or change.
3 The cost of the development or change. The provider ought to analyse these costs between:
   (a) *variable costs*, i.e. costs that increase or decrease with every activity change, for example, consumable items;
   (b) *additional staffing or semi-fixed costs*, i.e. the numbers and grades of staff required and the additional activity levels that this number of staff could provide, before more staff are required;
   (c) *any new equipment or building adaptations* that are required in order for the development/change to take place, i.e. the capital costs of the development. The business case should also show the number of years over which the capital investment will be written off, i.e. the standard life of the building or equipment.
4 Where possible, some indication from the main purchasers that they have shown a commitment to the proposed development or change.
5 The financial break-even point of the proposal. This is important for all managers as it is an indication of the financial risk involved in the development. For example, if the price charged to the purchasers equates exactly to the annual running costs of the development or change, there is no room for a price reduction should another provider offer the same service at a lower price to the purchasers. Under this scenario, you may be forced to reduce your price and would have to undertake more activity in order to break even. Knowledge of the likely competition and, therefore, the price sensitivity is crucial to any business development.
6 The key contacts for purchasers in relation to the development or change. This is particularly relevant for general practitioners, be they fundholders or not, who often, when a new service is developed, would like to speak to the lead clinician and be clear about the referral routes into the new service etc. or actually visit the hospital department involved in the development and see how things work in

practice. As providers move more and more into marketing their services, it becomes increasingly important to be 'customer friendly' and the starting point is often in the well-presented business case.

When a new development or service change is agreed between purchasers and providers, it is important to remember that the overall contractual commitment of the provider to the purchasers has been influenced and the formal contracts should be amended accordingly for monitoring services. The contract adjustments would be:

1 potential increase in contract activity;
2 an increase in hospital costs, therefore, an increase in the contract price;
3 an improvement in the quality of patient care which may be able to be set into new standards for monitoring purposes.

In summary, the process for developing services or changing clinical practice in the new National Health Service will follow a pathway as described below:

1 Develop a business case along the lines described above.
↓
2 Ensure that the business case is approved by senior managers within the Trust or DMU.
↓
3 Finalise agreements with purchaser(s), in respect of the new development and amend contracts accordingly.
↓
4 Advise GPs of the service launch and referral process.
↓
5 Commence the service.
↓
6 Monitor activity, income and quality standards against those set out in the business case.

7

Conservative management of stress and urge incontinence

Jo Laycock

Introduction

Previously considered a soft option for the management of female urinary incontinence, conservative management has recently received many favourable reports in medical journals. Furthermore, development of a multi-disciplinary approach in many centres has led to physiotherapists and nurses incorporating bladder training and pelvic floor re-education in their treatment strategies. The use of biofeedback, perineometry and electrical stimulation is still the domain of the specialist physiotherapist, although these pelvic floor muscle (PFM) re-education modalities are incorporated in some specialist nurse treatment programmes in the USA.

Background

Stress incontinence may be due to urethral hypermobility and/or low urethral closure pressures. The result of a sudden increase in intra-abdominal pressure (such as coughing) can, therefore, produce poor transmission of pressure to the proximal urethra and/or inadequate compensatory increase in urethral closure pressure. Both these scenarios may cause incontinence and both may be remedied by increasing the contractility of the pelvic floor muscles.

Urge incontinence occurs when a patient is unable to inhibit a detrusor contraction in the filling phase of the micturition cycle. A number of inhibitory reflexes govern this control including the resting and active contractility of the pelvic floor muscles (Mahoney *et al.* 1980).

Pelvic floor muscles

The medial portion of the levator ani is concerned with maintaining continence, and is a heterogeneous mixture of slow- and fast-twitch muscle fibres. The slow-twitch fibres are responsible for the postural response and the fast-twitch fibres are recruited (reflexly) during coughing, sneezing, etc. Obstetric trauma, resulting in muscle damage and partial denervation (with subsequent re-innervation) has been demonstrated in 80% of primiparous women (Allen *et al.* 1990) and is generally considered a causative factor in pelvic floor dysfunction leading to urinary incontinence. Cortical awareness of pelvic floor contractility may be lost due to pain and trauma in childbirth and the result of incomplete re-innervation; consequently, a weak pelvic floor may result. However, many women do not present with incontinence until later in life and this may be attributed to further deterioration of muscle tone due to the ageing process and hormonal changes in the menopause. Other factors associated with weak PFM include constipation and obesity.

Muscle training

Three basic principles of muscle training should be applied to a lax pelvic floor to ensure a training effect; namely, overload, specificity and reversibility. Overload implies the need to exercise muscles up to their maximum capability and to ensure progression of time and effort as contractility improves. Specificity demands specific exercises for the slow- and fast-twitch muscle fibres and functional training. For example, patients are taught to contract their PFM before and during a cough or when lifting. Reversibility refers to the need to continue to exercise as a life-long habit to prevent a return to the weakened state.

Pelvic floor assessment

Digital palpation by the examining health professional, be it gynaecologist, physiotherapist, nurse or GP will identify the correct pelvic floor muscle contraction. However, over 30% of women are unable to perform a voluntary contraction and require special tuition. Instruction to squeeze on the examiner's finger(s) and to tighten the PFM as if preventing the passing of flatus, helps the patient to understand the correct action, and the power of the muscle is determined by pressure on the examiner's finger(s). This can be followed by a simple (pressure) perineometric assessment (Figure 7.1); however, many patients concomitantly contract their abdominals and this may produce a false perineometer reading.

Pelvic floor exercises

Patient specific pelvic floor exercises (PFE) are a series of maximum muscle contractions aimed at training the levator ani to contract with increasing power and endurance and to provide increased resting tone. They should be practised several times a day and the patient advised that treatment may take three to six months, depending on their compliance to the home exercise programme and the level of pelvic laxity present.

Results

Reported results of pelvic floor re-education vary depending on the methodology of assessing outcomes. Ideally, both objective measures (pad test, urethral pressures) and subjective measures should be adopted in assessing surgery, drug therapy and physiotherapy, and until these are standardised, it will always be difficult to compare clinical outcomes. However, within these limitations, Sandri *et al.* (1988) reported

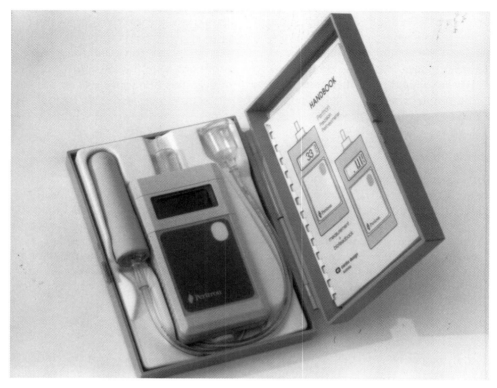

Figure 7.1   Peritron. Pressure sensitive perineometer for assessment of pelvic floor muscle contractility

on a study of 24 women with genuine stress incontinence (mean age 50) treated with pelvic floor exercises. Objectively they demonstrated that 65% were essentially dry after treatment, and subjectively reported 12% unchanged, 12% slightly improved, 35% markedly improved and 41% cured. A further study by Shaikh *et al.* (1993) (n = 20; age 19–77 years) reported that 60% of women demonstrated a significant improvement in urethral closure pressures and subjectively, 50% were cured with a further 30% much improved.

The success of PFE depends on the motivation and enthusiasm of both the patient and the health professionals prescribing and overseeing the treatment.

Vaginal cones

Weight training for the pelvic floor muscles was introduced by Plevnik in 1985. A cone is placed in the vagina above the pelvic floor, and the feeling of loosing the cone encourages the woman to contract her pelvic floor to retain it. Available in

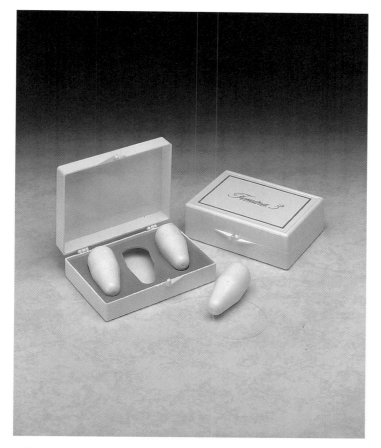

Figure 7.2 Femina Cones

sets of three numbered cones increasing in weight (see Figure 7.2) the cones are used first in standing, progressing to walking, jumping and coughing.

Results

Peattie *et al.* (1988) took 30 women (age 18–47) from the waiting list for surgery and treated them with cone therapy, reporting 70% cured or improved, and 63% declining surgery. However, Kondo *et al.* (1993) (n = 45; age 28–76) reported clinical success in only 13% of their patients, with 17% unable to retain even the lightest cone.

Biofeedback

Biofeedback translates PFM activity into a more understandable event, which has been shown to improve both muscular effort and co-ordination. This can be supplied using a simple pressure perineometer or sophisticated computer-driven pressure or EMG monitoring via vaginal or anal probes.

Results

Burgio *et al.* (1985) gave four weeks of twice weekly biofeedback to 14 women with stress incontinence using sophisticated instrumental visual and auditory feedback. They demonstrated 79% subjective reduction in incontinence and a significant ($p<0.05$) increase in sphincter strength, compared with a control group of women ($n=11$) treated by digital palpation and verbal feedback, who showed 51% reduction in incontinence and no significant improvement in sphincter strength.

   Woolmer (1994) reported symptomatic relief of patients presenting with interstitial cystitis and/or detrusor instability, pain, incontinence and frequency. Symptoms were greatly reduced by bladder training and teaching control of the pelvic floor muscles.

Electrical stimulation

Neuromuscular electrical stimulation (NMS) is widely used in the management of both stress and urge incontinence. For incontinent women with a weak pelvic floor, application of a maximum current is said to provide artificial muscle exercise and to 'facilitate' voluntary control by providing the 'feeling' of PFM contraction. Furthermore, a low-intensity, low-frequency current is reported to have a 'trophic' effect on neuromuscular activity, enhancing the blood supply and encouraging muscle protein synthesis. All types of NMS are thought to encourage axonal sprouting and so improve re-innervation. Maximum intensity, low-frequency NMS applied to patients with urge incontinence has been shown to reduce both the frequency and magnitude of unstable detrusor contractions, by normalising reflex activity (Eriksen *et al.* 1989).

Results

Laycock and Jerwood (1993) compared transcutaneous interferential therapy ($n=23$) with pelvic floor exercises ($n=23$). There was no significant difference between the two groups: subjectively, 61% of the stimulation group and 41% of the PFE group were much improved or cured, and objectively 41% of the stimulation group and 60% of the PFE group demonstrated much improvement or cure (pad test). However, the transcutaneous method of application has been superseded in many centres by internal (vaginal/anal) electrodes which are reported to produce an enhanced clinical effect.

   Plevnik *et al.* (1986) treated 310 patients with mixed symptoms, using a home simulator for 30 days; 56% reported to be cured or improved, classified as satisfied with the treatment and not requesting any further intervention.

Summary

The clinical trials described in the text evaluated each modality in isolation. However, in clinical practice, biofeedback and NMS are adjuncts to pelvic floor exercises and combination therapy is generally the treatment of choice.

   The results of conservative management of GSI do not compete with surgery, but the outcomes reported herein justify further research to determine the optimum treatment (or combination treatment) and the patients most likely to benefit from this approach.

References

Allen, R.E., Hosker, G.L., Smith, A.R.B. and Warrell, D.W. (1990) Pelvic floor damage and childbirth: a neurophysiological study. *Br J Obstet Gynaecol* **97**, 770–9

Burgio, K.L., Robinson, J.C. and Engel, B.T. (1986) The role of biofeedback in Kegel exercise training for stress urinary incontinence. *Am J Obstet Gynecol* **154**, 58–64

Eriksen, B. *et al.* (1989) Maximal electrostimulation of the pelvic floor in female idiopathic destrusor instability and urge incontinence. *Neurourol Urodyn* **8**, 219–30

Kondo, A. *et al.* (1989) Prospective analysis of the vaginal cone treatment for stress incontinence. *ICS (Rome)* (suppl.) 133

Laycock, J. and Jerwood, D. (1993) Does pre-modulated interferential therapy cure genuine stress incontinence? *Physiotherapy* **79**, 553–60

Mahoney, D.T. *et al.* (1980) Incontinence of urine due to instability of micturition reflexes. Part 1. Urology, XV 3: 229–239 Part 2. Urology, XV 4: 379–88

Peattie, A.B., Plevnik, S. and Stanton, S.L. (1988) Vaginal cones: a conservative method of treating genuine stress incontinence. *Br J Obstet Gynaecol* **95**, 1049–53

Plevnik, S. *et al.* (1986) Short term electrical stimulation: home treatment for urinary incontinence. *World J Urol* **4**, 24–6

Sandri, S.D. *et al.* (1986) Pad controlled results of pelvic floor physiotherapy in female stress incontinence. *Proceedings of ICS Boston*, pp. 233–5

Shaikh, N., Mordey, S., Morris, J. and Arkell, D. (1993) An objective assessment of pelvic physiotherapy: female stress incontinence. *ICS (Rome)* (suppl.) 209–10

Woolmer, B. (1994) in J. Laycock and J.J. Wyndaele (Eds) *Understanding the Pelvic Floor.* Dereham: Neen House Books

8

Anterior repair

A. R. B. Smith

Introduction

Until the development and popularisation of the abdominal approach to anterior vaginal wall prolapse by Marshall *et al.* (1949) and Burch (1961), anterior vaginal repair was the standard approach to the surgical management of cystocele and stress incontinence of urine. More recently the concept of surgical repair of fascial defects including midline, lateral and transverse tears in the fascia, has been revived, suggesting that there may be a place for anterior repair in selected cases.

Birth of the anterior vagina repair

George White, an American surgeon, first reported on the paravaginal repair for the cure of cystocele in 1909 (White 1909). He used two lateral anterior vaginal wall incisions to gain access to the pubovesical fascia and the arcus tendineus levator ani from under the subpubic arch to the ischial spine posteriorly. White acknowledged that the procedure could be performed abdominally through the retropubic space, but felt that a vaginal approach was preferable. In 1913 Howard Kelly, a pioneer of gynaecological surgery in the USA, described the technique of midline fascial plication, including the Kelly stitch under the urethrovesical junction, for the correction of stress incontinence of urine (Kelly 1913). It is fair to say that Kelly's approach of midline fascial plication gained greater acceptance than the paravaginal repair partly because of it being a simpler concept and partly because of ease of the surgical procedure.

Alternative approaches to surgery

Dissatisfaction with the frequency of recurrence of stress incontinence and encouraging results from retropubic approaches to bladder neck surgery by Marshall *et al.* (1949) and Burch (1961) led many gynaecologists and urologists to reappraise their surgical management. Many continue to employ the Kelly type anterior repair as a first-line procedure before employing the retropubic/abdominal approach for recurrence (Hilton 1990). Others, in recognising that most studies indicate that the first procedure has the greatest chance of success, have abandoned the anterior repair completely. Increasing concern has been expressed, however, about the higher incidence of post-operative voiding problems (Kiilholma *et al.* 1993), detrusor

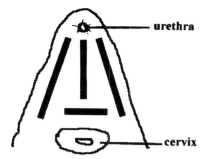

Figure 8.1 Sites of fascial defect in anterior vaginal wall

instability (Cardozo *et al.* 1979) and occurrence of vaginal prolapse needing surgery at a later date (Wiskind *et al.* 1992) following abdominal procedures. It is probable that the higher success rate in curing stress incontinence associated with greater bladder neck elevation will carry an inevitable increased morbidity in other areas of bladder function. In a retrospective review of 519 anterior repair procedures Beck *et al.* (1990) found stress incontinence was cured in 84% of selected cases with new detrusor instability demonstrated in 6% and significant morbidity excluding incontinence in only 1%. The study also highlighted the importance of placement of retropubic sutures to provide higher urethral support than is possible with a central Kelly type central plication. The technique could be interpreted as combining the operative techniques of White (1909) and Kelly (1913). Shull and Baden (1989) have demonstrated that, having first identified the fascial defect, be it lateral, longitudinal or transverse, the vaginal approach to repair can result in cure in 95% of cases. Park and Miller (1988) in a long-term follow-up of abdominal and vaginal bladder neck surgery demonstrated a parallel risk of recurrence with time, with all procedures. It would appear that whatever surgery is performed the effect of ageing and life events such as childbirth will contrive to increase the risk of recurrence.

Anterior repair technique

Important points

1 Identification of defects.
   Careful examination of the anterior vaginal wall will illustrate whether there is a central lateral or upper transverse defect or a combination of these (see Figure 8.1).
2 Midline anterior vaginal wall incision.
3 Identify pubovesical fascia and defects in fascia.
4 Repair defects with vicryl/dexon (catgut is probably inadequate). If lateral defects are identified fascia must be re-attached to arcus tendineus levator ani from under the subpubic arch to the ischial spine. Failure to identify a lateral defect is probably the most common cause for failure of the anterior repair.
5 Close vaginal wall.
6 Catheterise for approximately 48 hours. Voiding problems are rare since there should be no urethral obstruction produced by repair of fascial defects.

References

Beck, R.P., McCormick, S. and Nordstrum, L. (1990) 25-year experience with 519 anterior colporrhaphy procedures. *Obstet Gynecol* **78**, 1011–18

Burch, J.C. (1961) Urethrovaginal fixation to Cooper's ligament for correction of stress incontinence, cystocele and prolapse. *Am J Obstet Gynecol* **81**, 281–90

Cardozo, L.D., Stanton, S.L. and Williams, J.E. (1979) Detrusor instability following surgery for genuine stress incontinence. *Br J Urol* **51**, 204–7

Hilton, P. (1990) 'Surgery for genuine stress incontinence: which operation and for which patient?' in J.O. Drife, P. Hilton and S.L. Stanton (Eds) *Micturition.* Proceedings of the 21st RCOG Study Group, pp. 225–46. London: Springer-Verlag

Kelly, H.A. (1913) Incontinence of urine in women. *Urol Cutan Rev* **17**, 291

Kiilholma, P., Makinen, J., Chancellor, M.B. *et al.* (1993) Modified Burch colposuspension for stress urinary incontinence in females. *Surgery, Gynecology and Obstetrics* **176**, 111–15

Marshall, V.F., Marchetti, A.A. and Krantz, K.E. (1949) The correction of stress incontinence by simple vesicourethral suspension. *Surgery, Gynecology and Obstetrics* **88**, 509–18

Park, E.S. and Miller, E.J. (1988) Surgical treatment of stress urinary incontinence: a comparison of the Kelly plication, Marshall–Marchetti–Krantz and Pereyra procedures. *Obstet Gynecol* **71**, 575–9

Shull, B.L. and Baden, W.F. (1989) A six year experience with paravaginal defect repair. *Am J Obstet Gynecol* **160**, 1432–40

White, G.R. (1909) Cystocele. *JAMA* **103**, 21, 1707–10

Wiskind, A.K., Creighton, S.M. and Stanton, S.L. (1992) The incidence of genital prolapse after the Burch colposuspension. *Am J Obstet Gynecol* **167**, 399–405

9

Colposuspension in the treatment of genuine stress incontinence

Paul Hilton

Introduction

Genuine stress incontinence is defined as the involuntary loss of urine through an intact urethra, when the intravesical pressure exceeds the maximum urethral pressure in the absence of detrusor contraction. Typically patients complain of the symptom of stress incontinence, i.e. urine leakage on exertion, and the clinical sign of stress incontinence is demonstrable on pelvic examination. Since the first description of a suprapubic cystotomy by Baker-Brown in 1864, over 100 different operations have been described for the treatment of stress incontinence. The vaginal approach remains the most widely employed procedure undertaken by gynaecologists, although of the suprapubic procedures, the colposuspension is increasing in popularity (Hilton 1990). The original description of the operation, then called the urethro-vaginal suspension was by Burch in 1961; several modifications to the technique, and terminology, have been employed, the term colposuspension being coined by Turner-Warwick and Whiteside in 1970.

Indications and contraindications

The main indication for colposuspension is of course in the surgical treatment of symptomatic stress incontinence. Predisposing or precipitating factors should have been excluded or remedied first, conservative treatments should have been attempted, and ideally urodynamic investigation undertaken to confirm the diagnosis of genuine stress incontinence. The significance of vaginal prolapse in the role of colposuspension is argued; whilst many gynaecologists look on the operation as inappropriate where there is cystourethrocele, it was actually in the management of combined stress incontinence with prolapse that Burch first described the procedure.

It has become accepted wisdom that in the face of known detrusor instability conventional bladder neck elevating procedures should be considered contraindicated. Several studies have shown the results to be less satisfactory in this situation, although more recent work has suggested that with low pressure unstable contractions reasonable success may be achieved. Provided stress incontinence is a major factor in the symptomatology, attempts have been made to stabilise the bladder first, and the patient accepts that the associated symptoms of frequency and urgency may remain or even deteriorate, detrusor instability should no longer be looked on as an absolute contraindication to colposuspension, or other procedures.

Voiding dysfunction should be seen as a relative contraindication. The procedure is known to be associated with an increase in voiding pressure and decrease in urine flow rate post-operatively, and in those patients with abnormal voiding patterns pre-operatively, the result may be a clinically significant degree of obstruction. In some women this may be an acceptable risk, but it is preferable to teach such patients clean intermittent self catheterisation before carrying out surgery; alternatively, a less obstructive procedure might be considered.

The procedure appears to be effective by elevating the bladder neck into a high retropubic position, thus increasing the transmission of intra-abdominal pressure rises to the proximal urethra. In patients whose bladder neck is already well elevated, therefore, it is unlikely that colposuspension (or other elevating procedures for that matter) will achieve much improvement. Similarly, marked narrowing, or shortening of the vagina, or immobility from previous surgical scarring or radiation etc. may mean that adequate elevation is unlikely to result.

As a general rule for all continence operations, it is wise that the patient should have completed her family beforehand. Further pregnancy may itself result in deterioration in continence, and vaginal delivery should certainly be looked on as contraindicated in patients who reach the end of pregnancy still symptom-free.

Obesity and chronic respiratory problems have often been looked on as contraindications to incontinence surgery. Experience suggests that obese patients rarely lose weight prior to surgery however; and although the post-operative morbidity may be increased, the results of colposuspension are as good in the obese as those of normal weight (Stanton 1986).

Procedure

Pre-operative evaluation

Pre-operative evaluation should include a clinical assessment as to the appropriateness and feasibility of the procedure, in particular in relation to the degree of elevation of the bladder neck, and the capacity and mobility of the vagina. The pelvic organs as a whole should be assessed, and the need for any additional gynaecological surgery considered. If a significant degree of uterine descent is present, hysterectomy should be carried out simultaneously. Similarly, if there is enterocele or rectocele, even if asymptomatic, these are probably best dealt with at the time of colposuspension, by colposacropexy or perineorrhaphy; if not they will almost certainly require further intervention shortly thereafter. Ideally urodynamic investigation should be carried out, to confirm the diagnosis of genuine stress incontinence, and to exclude or evaluate the presence of coexisting detrusor instability or voiding dysfunction. Whilst neither would absolutely contraindicate the operation, their presence would undoubtedly influence pre-operative counselling.

Preparation

No special pre-operative preparation is required, except for abdominal and perineal shave. Subcutaneous heparin is recommended for prophylaxis against deep vein thrombosis, and some surgeons advocate antibiotic prophylaxis. General or regional anaesthesia are equally appropriate, and a modified lithotomy position, using Lloyd-Davies stirrups is preferred.

Operative technique

The following section describes the author's own version of the procedure; this is covered in greater depth in Hilton (1987).

1 The abdomen, vagina and perineum are cleansed and draped, a plastic transurethral resection drape being used for the perineum, thus allowing access to the vagina by way of the sterile condom.

2 A Foley catheter is left on free drainage throughout the procedure.

3 A low transverse suprapubic incision is made no more than 1 cm above the pubic symphysis, so as to gain optimum access to the retropubic space. Cherney's modification, separating the recti from their insertion onto the symphysis may improve access in some circumstances. After incising and freeing the rectus sheath, the rectus and pyramidalis muscles are separated in the midline and freed from the underlying bladder and peritoneum.

4 A Millin bladder retractor is preferred, the blades taking up relatively little room in the incision in comparison to the four bladed ring retractor advocated by some authors.

5 The bladder and urethra are freed from the back of the symphysis and obturator internus fascia. This is usually easily achieved by blunt finger dissection, although where there has been previous retropubic surgery, sharp dissection should be used.

6 Having opened up the retropubic space, the operator (assuming him to be right-handed and standing to the patient's left side) introduces the index finger of the left hand into the vagina, maintaining sterility using the sterile transurethral resection drape. The finger presses against one or other antero-lateral vaginal wall, to elevate a cone of tissue, not as is often supposed in the lateral fornix, but within the lower 4–5 cm of the vagina, alongside the bladder neck.

7 Whilst maintaining upward and lateral pressure from below, the operator uses his other hand to reflect the bladder and bladder neck medially off the underlying fascia. In previously unoperated cases this is usually achieved easily by blunt dissection aided by a swab on a sponge-holding forcep, or a small 'cherry' swab mounted on a Meig's forcep (see Figure 9.1). Where there has been previous surgery sharp dissection may be required. Many veins of the vesical plexus may be encountered during the dissection; larger ones should be controlled by diathermy or ligation, but smaller vessels are usually easily controlled by maintaining pressure from below until the suspension sutures are tied.

8 The paravaginal fascia should be identified as a white glistening layer from the level of the bladder neck, up to the apex of the cone elevated by the vaginal finger; this may therefore be a variable length, depending on the extent of vaginal wall descent. Once cleared, sutures are inserted into the fascia, starting at the bladder neck, and working upwards and lateral along the bladder base. Usually three sutures approximately 1 cm apart are sufficient, although more may be used where there is a large cystocele. Either a slowly absorbable suture such as

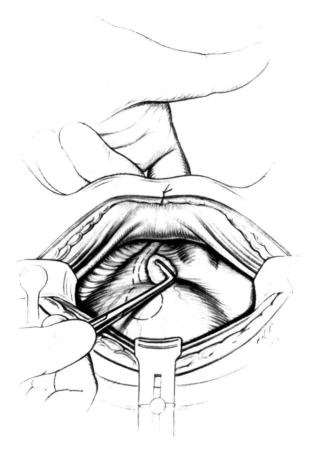

Figure 9.1 The paravaginal fascia alongside the bladder neck is elevated by the operator's finger from below; the bladder is then reflected medially off the fascia, to ensure safe and accurate suture placement. (From Hilton (1987) with permission from the publisher.)

polyglactin (Vicryl) where the vagina comes easily in to apposition with the iliopectineal ligament, or a non-absorbable (Ethibond) where there is any degree of bow-stringing should be used. As each suture is inserted into the fascia it is tied, first to aid haemostasis, and second to avoid the stitch running when it is later tied to the ligament. The suture is then secured to the most adjacent portion of the iliopectineal ligament. For the lowermost sutures this may not be possible without some degree of bow-stringing, and in this situation it is preferable to hitch the stitch to the periosteum of the pubis before securing to lacunar ligament. The second and third sutures are similarly inserted, but should easily be located into the iliopectineal ligament itself. A dry swab is left in place alongside the sutures to control any venous bleeding, and the dissection and suturing then undertaken on the other side.

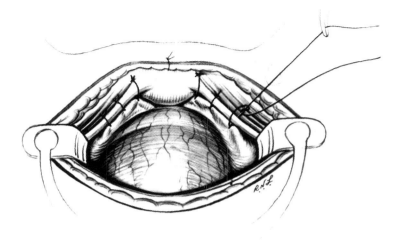

Figure 9.2   The sutures are tied up alternating sides; if tension is put on the suture limb through the ligament, the vagina is brought into apposition with the ligament without the need for pressure from below. (From Hilton (1987) with permission from the publisher.)

9 Once all six sutures are in place they are then tied up alternating sides, starting from the lowermost suture on one side and finishing with the uppermost on the other side. By putting tension on the suture limb through the ligament, the fascia and underlying vaginal wall are brought into proximity to the ligament without the need for pressure from below (see Figure 9.2).

10 Suction drainage should be used in the retropubic space, and suprapubic catheterisation is recommended for ease of post-operative management.

If vaginal examination is undertaken immediately post-operatively the vagina should be found to be extremely well elevated, with the external meatus pulled round beneath the symphysis (see Figure 9.3). A crescentic web is also often evident on the posterior vaginal wall, where the pre-rectal fascia is pulled forward; by the time of outpatient review this has usually resolved, whilst the bladder neck remains supported.

Post-operative management

Heparin should be continued until the patient is fully mobile; if prophylactic antibiotics are used, no more than 48 hours would be required. Urine cultures are checked every 48 hours, but in the absence of fever asymptomatic infection probably does not require treatment. Suction drains can usually be removed after 24–36 h.

The catheter is clamped on the third day, and the residual volume checked in the evening unless the patient is unable to void or becomes uncomfortable. Once the patient is voiding volumes greater than 200 ml, with an evening residual volume less

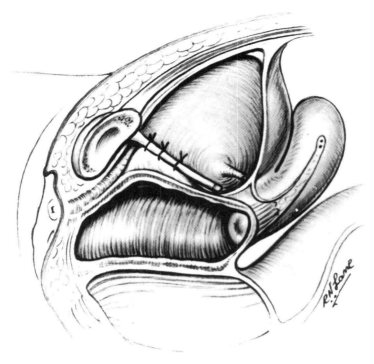

Figure 9.3   Vaginal examination confirms the degree of elevation of the bladder neck immediately post-operatively. (From Hilton (1987) with permission from the publisher.)

than 100 ml, the catheter is clamped overnight; if the residual the next morning is less than 100 ml the catheter is left clamped for a full 24 h, and if the residual thereafter is low, the catheter is removed and the patient discharged.

Complications

Operative

Intra-operative complications include haemorrhage from perivesical veins, injury to the bladder or urethra, and ureteric damage. Recognised injury to the bladder or urethra should be repaired with one or two layers of 2/0 absorbable suture; effective drainage should be ensured, using a wide bore catheter, and maintained for at least five days. If hysterectomy has been carried out simultaneously, or there is other continuity with the vagina, 10–12 days' drainage would be advised.

Injury to the ureters is fortunately uncommon, but ligation may occur if care is not taken to identify the paravaginal fascia clearly. On occasion, especially where there is a large degree of cystocele and additional sutures are inserted, distortion of the bladder base in the region of the uretero-vesical junction may result in kinking of the ureter with consequent obstruction; it is unlikely that this would be recognised at operation and is more likely to present in the early post-operative period with loin pain or fever.

Early

Where ureteric obstruction as above is suspected this should be investigated as a matter of urgency, by IVU or renal ultrasound, with isotope renography to assess relative function; this should be followed by retrograde pyelography. If ureteric stenting can be achieved either retrogradely or via a percutaneous nephrostomy, then drainage with a double pig-tail stent for a period of months may allow complete resolution of the problem; otherwise laparotomy and ureteric re-implantation would be necessary.

Other complications of the early post-operative period include urinary tract infection, thrombo-embolic complications, retropubic or wound haematoma and infection, and delay in resumption of spontaneous micturition. The latter might be considered to be present when the patient is unable to void by seven days following surgery, and is reported in 12–25% of patients. Although various drug treatments have been advocated, the optimum management is to discharge the patient with a suprapubic catheter *in situ*, once they are happy to manage it (i.e. clamp, release, and check residual volumes). They will usually be able to void more freely in the privacy of their home, and if reviewed a week later, catheter removal can be undertaken, having ensured that the residual is less than 100 ml, on the same criteria as detailed above for in-patient management.

To some extent the problems of delayed voiding may be predicted from pre-operative urodynamic investigation. Patients voiding by valsalva manoeuvre, or with a low pressure, low-flow voiding pattern or those with a poor or absent isometric detrusor contraction have been reported to be at increased risk of such problems.

Late

Voiding dysfunction is also perhaps one of the commonest complications in the longer term following colposuspension, although it is not necessarily those patients with immediate post-operative difficulties who also have late problems. Several studies have shown the procedure to be consistently associated with an increase in voiding pressure, and a decrease in urine flow rate, and 10–20% of patients may develop a significant degree of outflow obstruction. It has been shown that voiding difficulty is associated with extreme elevation and reduced mobility of the bladder neck post-operatively.

Other long-term complications include the development of detrusor instability, uterine or vault prolapse, and dyspareunia. Detrusor instability has been reported following most bladder neck elevating operations; it tends to be more common following the more obstructive procedures, and may be seen in up to 20% of patients (Cardozo *et al.* 1979). Such cases tend to be particularly resistant to treatment, approximately 60% remaining symptomatic at 3–5 years following surgery (Steele *et al.* 1985).

Several studies have alluded to the development of uterine or vault prolapse following colposuspension, and prevalence figures of between 6 and 17% have been reported. No control data exist, however, and whether this represents a significant increase is difficult to judge. It is as well to remember that patients with stress incontinence may have both neuromuscular and connective tissue defects contributing to their pathology, and it should not be surprising that they subsequently develop additional pelvic floor problems in other areas in significant numbers. It is possible that the relocation of the bladder neck into a high retropubic position encourages intra-abdominal pressure changes to be directed more towards the vault, with subsequent increased tendency to enterocele development. Wiskind *et al.* (1992) reported that 27% of patients following colposuspension required further prolapse surgery, and certainly where any evidence of vault or posterior wall prolapse exists at the time of assessment of stress incontinence it is wise to consider additional procedures to correct this at the time of initial surgery.

Dyspareunia is reported by some patients at the time of initial follow-up. This seems most often due to mechanical problems as a result of the crescentic ridge of pre-rectal fascia pulled forward at operation. This usually settles with 6–8 weeks of surgery, and patients are best advised to refrain from coitus during this period. Urinary leakage specifically during intercourse is a surprisingly common occurrence among incontinent women, but on occasion may be noted for the first time following colposuspension. This probably reflects the mechanism by which the operation alters bladder neck position and function (Hilton and Stanton 1983; Hertogs and Stanton 1985). Although varying urodynamic findings may be found, the problem is best managed by encouraging complete voiding, or even clean intermittent self catheterisation, immediately prior to intercourse.

Results

Evaluation of the results of surgical studies is difficult for several reasons: the duration and completeness of follow-up may vary; authors employ widely varying criteria for success, some being entirely subjective, others objective; even those with objective outcome measures, may differ in the variables used, some bearing little relevance to clinical results.

Not withstanding these difficulties the results of colposuspension have been consistently good, with cure rates between 70 and 100% reported. In the recent meta-analysis of surgical results by Jarvis (1994) involving a total of 213 studies, 89.6% (n = 1726) were subjectively cured, and 84.3% (n = 2300) objectively cured by colposuspension. As found previously by others, the results of primary surgery were better than those with previous unsuccessful operations, at 89.8% and 82.5% respectively.

Most surgical studies report success in terms of relieving the symptom of stress incontinence. Although as above, some patients may develop symptomatic detrusor for the first time following surgery, it has been shown that, of those with mixed symptoms before operation, approximately one third will find their frequency, urgency or urge incontinence improved following colposuspension.

Causes of failure

Surgery in general, and colposuspension in particular, may be unsuccessful for a variety of reasons. Detrusor instability may become apparent, either having been present but undiagnosed previously, or developing *de novo* following the procedure. Voiding dysfunction, with a persistent residual volume may result in overflow incontinence, not readily distinguishable by the patient from the stress incontinence with which she presented.

More often lack of success with colposuspension is due to failure to achieve adequate elevation of the bladder neck. This may reflect either technical failure, or poor case selection. The operation is ill-chosen if the vaginal capacity and mobility are inadequate, since good approximation of the paravaginal fascia to the iliopectineal ligaments is unlikely to result. Alternatively if the bladder neck is already elevated, but the urethra itself inherently weak, an elevating procedure could not be deemed appropriate, since further elevation is unlikely to be beneficial; in this latter group urethral reconstruction, artificial sphincter, or periurethral injections are probably more appropriate operations.

References

Burch, J. (1961) Urethrovaginal fixation to Cooper's ligament for correction of stress incontinence, cystocele and prolapse. *Am J Obstet Gynecol* **81**, 281–90

Cardozo, L.D., Stanton, S.L. and Williams, J. (1979) Detrusor instability following surgery for genuine stress incontinence. *Br J Obstet Gynaecol* **51**, 204–7

Hertogs, K. and Stanton, S.L. (1985) Mechanism of continence after colposuspension. *Br J Urol* **92**, 1184–8

Hilton, P. and Stanton, S.L. (1983) A clinical and urodynamic evaluation of the Burch colposuspension for genuine stress incontinence. *Br J Obstet Gynaecol* **90**, 934–9

Hilton, P. (1987) 'Surgery for urinary stress incontinence' in J. Monaghan (Ed.) *Rob and Smith's Operative Surgery: Gynaecology and Obstetrics* (4th ed.), pp. 105–26. London: Chapman and Hall

Hilton, P. (1990) 'Surgery for genuine stress incontinence: which operation and for which patient?' in J.O. Drife, P. Hilton and S.L. Stanton (Eds) *Micturition. Proceedings of the 21st RCOG Study Group*, pp. 225–46. London: Springer-Verlag

Jarvis, G. (1994) Surgery for genuine stress incontinence. *Br J Obstet Gynaecol* **101**, 371–4

Stanton, S.L. (1986) 'Colposuspension' in S.L. Stanton and E.A. Tanagho (Eds) *Surgery for Female Incontinence* (2nd ed.), pp. 95–103. London and Berlin: Springer-Verlag

Steele, S.A., Cox, C. and Stanton, S.L. (1985) Long-term follow-up of detrusor instability following the colposuspension operation. *Br J Urol* **58**, 138–42

Turner-Warwick, R. and Whiteside, G. (1970) 'Investigation and management of bladder neck dysfunction' in E. Riches (Ed.) *Modern Trends in Urology*, pp. 295–311. London: Butterworth

Wiskind, A.K., Creighton, S.M. and Stanton, S.L. (1992) The incidence of genital prolapse after the Burch colposuspension. *Am J Obstet Gynecol* **167**, 399–405

10

The Stamey operation for genuine stress incontinence of urine

William T. Lawrence

While the common aim of surgery for genuine stress incontinence is to elevate and support the bladder neck tissues, the type of operation and route chosen for the repair has largely depended on the training of the surgeon and the severity of the anatomical abnormality. Vaginal repairs have principally been the domain of gynaecologists, while open suprapubic colposuspensions have been performed by both gynaecologists and urologists.

Having recognised the advantages of the suprapubic approach to bladder neck surgery described by Marshall *et al.* (1949), Pereyra (1959) described a simplified bladder neck suspension procedure. The original procedure involved the passage of a long needle with an eye near its point blindly through the vaginal wall lateral to the bladder neck on each side. The steel wire suture was tied over the rectus sheath through two small lateral suprapubic incisions. With a modified technique incorporating an absorbable suture and an anterior vaginal repair Pereyra and Lebhertz (1967) reported an initial success rate of 94% which fell to 84% with longer follow-up. Pereyra attributed the recurrence of stress incontinence to failure of the absorbable suture, but recognised that a non-absorbable suture can fail by cutting through fascia. To try to avoid cut-through by suture material Pereyra and Lebhertz (1978) further modified the procedure by incorporating a helical suture into the periurethral fascia. With this modification an 87% success rate for primary surgery was reported on four-year follow-up.

Further interest developed in needle colposuspension when Stamey (1973) described a modification of the Pereyra procedure incorporating a Dacron buffer into the periurethral suture to prevent the suture cutting through the fascia (Figure 10.1). Stamey also recommended cystoscopy during the procedure to prevent bladder injury during needle placement. In a series of 203 patients Stamey (1980) reported a 91% cure rate, but long-term review was not included in many patients. Hilton and Mayne (1991) reported on a series of 100 women with up to four years follow-up of the Stamey procedure. At three months follow-up the objective cure rate was 83%, but at four years was 53% in patients under 65 years and 76% in older patients. Hilton and Mayne (1991) suggested that reduced activity in the elderly may be responsible for the higher success rate. Peattie and Stanton (1989) reported an objective cure rate of only 41% in a group of 44 women following the Stamey operation. Hilton and Mayne (1991) found that pre-operative maximum urethral closure pressure did not appear to influence surgical outcome, but successful

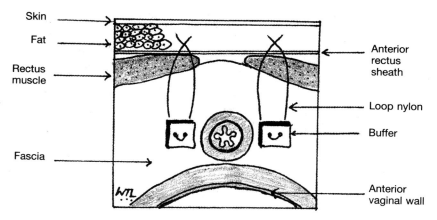

Skin

Fat

Rectus muscle

Fascia

Anterior rectus sheath

Loop nylon

Buffer

Anterior vaginal wall

Figure 10.1   Position of Stamey sutures

procedures were associated with enhancement of pressure transmission to the proximal quarters of the functional urethral length. It is not known whether the failure to provide adequate urethral support was through operative failure or post-operative failure.

The long-term success of the Stamey procedure has been shown to compare unfavourably to colposuspension. In a five-year follow-up of 127 women undergoing primary bladder neck surgery, Elia and Bergman (1994) reported a higher success rate for colposuspension than vaginal repair or Stamey procedure. Twice as many women were continent at five years following colposuspension than the vaginal repair or Stamey procedure (82% vs 37% and 43% respectively).

Patient selection

I have now performed several hundreds of these procedures and the principles which have attracted me to use this technique are that it is a dynamic operation. By that I mean that if the sutures are placed in the correct position and tied loosely the operation will work to support the bladder neck tissues during coughing, running, jumping or sneezing when extra strain is placed on the tissues. As the sutures are tied loosely there is very little post-operative voiding dysfunction compared with other operations for genuine stress incontinence.

The primary indication for the Stamey operation is for patients with genuine stress incontinence; and it is particularly suitable for patients who are obese or for those with a number of previous operative failures.

This operation has also been used successfully to tighten and elevate the bladder neck for patients with neurovesical dysfunction where prolonged catheterisation has caused urethral erosion. The aim of the operation for these patients is to maintain continence when leaving a suprapubic catheter in position, or to prevent recurrent urethral catheter extrusion.

The operation is also suitable for patients who have coexisting genuine stress incontinence and detrusor instability. The success rate for curing incontinence in these patients is not as high as for those with stress alone, and the instability must be amenable to treatment before embarking on surgery for sphincter weakness.

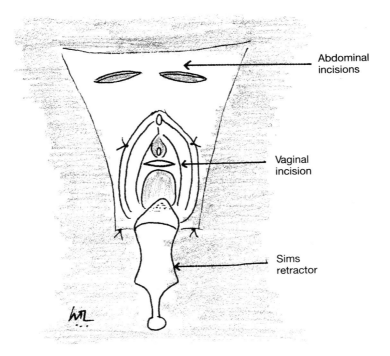

Figure 10.2   Sites of abdominal and vaginal incisions for Stamey colposuspension

The operation

Antibiotic prophylaxis is essential and a combination of Gentamicin and Metronidazole is satisfactory. Whenever possible, the Lloyd-Davis position is preferable; however, a useful alternative for patients with marked lower limb spasticity is a modified lithotomy position with knee crutches for leg support. Standard operative drapes are used, and it is advantageous to have a perineal tray for instruments during the vaginal dissection. It is important to exclude the anus from the operative field and this can be done simply by anchoring the towels with a silk stitch.

A weighted Sims speculum gives a good vaginal exposure, whereas an Auvard speculum is often too large. The special equipment required is a 'bladder neck suspension needle' for suture placement, and loop suture material and small buffers for vaginal anchoring.

Abdominal dissection

Two small suprapubic incisions (3–4 cm long) are made 4 cm above the pubic symphysis on each side of the midline (Figure 10.3). It is important that these incisions are high enough so that when they are deepened through superficial fat and Scarpa's fascia to the white layer of the rectus sheath the tied end of the loop suture will actually have some abdominal musculature to work with. If these sutures are tied very low near the pubic symphysis the operation will be less dynamic and this is certainly a cause for failure.

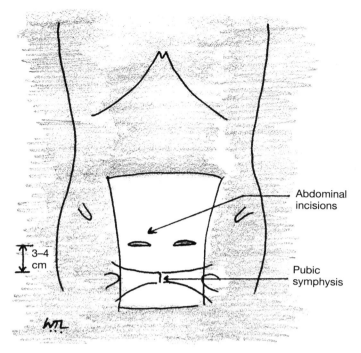

Figure 10.3   Position of abdominal incisions for Stamey colposuspension

Vaginal dissection

A preliminary cysto-urethroscopy is performed to exclude any unexpected bladder or urethral pathology (a 17 Ch scope and a 30° angle telescope lens are used). An 18 Ch Foley catheter is passed and the balloon filled with 20 ml of fluid. The urethra and bladder neck level are then readily identified by anterior vaginal palpation. After injecting a solution of local anaesthetic into the anterior vaginal wall, and up towards the bladder neck on each side, a transverse incision is made about 1 cm below the external urethral meatus. A plane can be developed close to the anterior vaginal wall by sharp scissor dissection.

When large enough, these developing para-urethral tunnels can be extended towards the bladder neck by a combination of blunt finger and scissor spreading dissection. Care must be taken to keep close to the anterior vaginal wall, otherwise the fascia may be weakened. Having reached the angle between the balloon and the shaft of the catheter, the mobilisation is repeated on the other side. Bleeding is never serious and can be easily controlled by a swab packing the vagina.

Needle placement

The needle can usually be used 'straight', but for very obese patients the malleable tip may be angled appropriately (Figure 10.4). There are three principal manoeuvres for needle placement:

1 With the needle held vertically at the medial end of one of the suprapubic incisions, it is advanced to pierce the rectus sheath. There is often a slight jerk as the needle passes through the sheath.

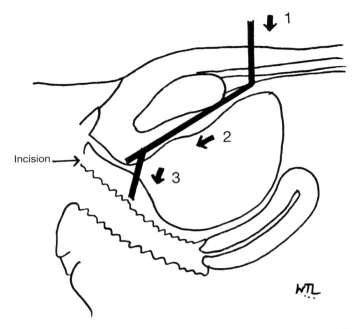

Figure 10.4   Placement of Stamey needle during colposuspension

2 The needle tip is immediately angled towards the top of the pubic bone to avoid
damage to deeper structures. By probing gently, the tip can be felt 'bouncing' on
the bone. (Obese patients with protruding abdominal tissue make it impossible to
do this with a straight needle and it is necessary to pre-bend the malleable tip.)
The needle is advanced down the back of the pubic bones for 1–2 cm. (When
operating on patients who have had previous open colposuspensions, the tip must
be kept very close to the bone, otherwise the needle will go though the bladder,
as this is often adherent to the pubic symphysis.)

   The index finger of one hand should then be placed up the appropriate bladder
neck tunnel. It is necessary to control the urethral catheter, either by palming it,
or getting an assistant to apply gentle traction, as necessary.

3 By slightly angling the needle tip downwards, it is readily palpated on the pulp
of the index finger. It is often necessary to withdraw the needle a little before
finally advancing it past the bladder neck in the angle of the catheter balloon and
shaft to appear from the vaginal incision below.

Endoscopic assessment

By gently moving the needle up and down while viewing the bladder neck with a 0°
or 30° telescope, it is possible to ensure that the medial stitch will be correctly
positioned. The tissues should move with the needle; if they do not, the needle is
too far lateral and can be withdrawn and repositioned. Side-to-side movement will
show if the needle is at the bladder neck level or too far down the urethra, which
may cause angulation of the urethra rather than elevation when the loops are tied.
The bladder is inspected on the anterior wall for needle perforation. This is usually

done with a 30° telescope, but if there is any doubt, a 70° lens will give a better view.

Positioning the loop sutures

One end of a loop suture is threaded through the needle aperture as it appears from the vaginal incision and this is drawn up to the abdomen. The bladder is emptied with a catheter and the needle passed from above a second time, 1.5–2 cm lateral to the medial stitch.

A small buffer already on the loop suture can be held with a 'Shod clamp' while the other end of the loop is drawn up with the second needle passage. The medial needle is positioned on the other side, and then a second cystoscopy can check this and the previous stitch. The bladder is emptied and the needle passed for the last time to complete the second loop. Gentle traction from above will guide the buffers up their respective paraurethral tunnels. A final cystoscopy will show the change in bladder neck configuration when gentle traction is applied. Movement can also be seen when looking at the anterior vaginal wall, and this gives some indication of how loose to tie the loops.

Vaginal wound closure

The vaginal incision is closed with a running mattress catgut stitch. It is important to ensure that the edges are everted and that no small blobs of fat protrude; these would form chronic granulations and predispose to infection. This incision must be closed before tying the loop sutures over the rectus sheath, because access for a good closure is lost when the bladder neck is drawn upwards.

Tying the loop sutures

The loop sutures should be tied with minimal tension, and if a general anaesthetic with muscle paralysis has been given, this should be taken into account, as the tissues will tighten up when the patient is awake. It is good practice to remove any vaginal speculum before tying the knots, because the weight can distort the tissues. Two throws (surgeon's knot) prevent any slipping and facilitate tying at the correct tension.

It should be possible to pass a fingertip underneath the knot, and, surprisingly, these are never too loose. If tied too tightly, however, it may be necessary to cut one stitch post-operatively. The suprapubic skin incisions may be closed with a subcuticular stitch.

The author has never used any buffer material in the abdominal incisions. This has been completely unnecessary and many abdominal buffers have been removed from other centres where infection has occurred. For some reason, at the present time unexplained, infection is more common in the abdominal incisions than the vaginal tunnels, though if the technique described is adhered to an infection rate of less than 1% can be expected.

Suprapubic catheterisation and post-operative care

Suprapubic drainage allows any periurethral oedema to settle and residual urine measurements may be easily taken. Some clinicians try clamping in the early post-operative period (2–5 days), but the author prefers to discharge patients home with the suprapubic catheter *in situ* 48 hours after surgery and re-admit them for voiding 8–12 days later. Although 70–80% of patients will void early, some will not, but after 10–14 days these patients can be encouraged to gently press suprapubically during voiding, which will allow a slight slacking of the loops, and so ease micturition. Approximately 99% of women will have no trouble at this time. Suprapubic catheterisation with an *Add-A-Cath* introducer is very satisfactory, allowing placement of a balloon catheter. No extra fixation with stitches is necessary, which is more comfortable for the patient and minimises infection.

Complications

Complications are few and are not serious. When inexperienced with the technique, there is a great temptation for the surgeon to tie the loops too tightly and this must be resisted. Excess tension may cause suprapubic pain post-operatively and the sutures will tend to 'cheese-wire' though the tissues. Voiding disorders are rare and the author's post-operative urodynamic measurements have not shown any outflow obstruction. Outflow obstruction has been reported, and it is associated with stitch tension. Urgency may be present post-operatively and can be treated with anticholinergic drugs. This may continue for several months in a few patients, but usually subsides. In cases of post-operative failure, a repeat Stamey procedure can be performed with good results.

Professor Stamey stated that 'the final evaluation of this procedure will, of course, have to wait for a later time and especially for the final arbiter of all successful surgical procedures – the experience of other surgeons who try it!' In my opinion, this is a good operation for 'surgically curable incontinence' and can be recommended for wider use in preference to colposuspension.

Equipment

Bladder neck suspension needles and *Add-A-Cath* suprapubic introducers may be obtained from Femcare Ltd, 67 St Peters Street, Nottingham NG7 3EN.

References

Elia, G. and Bergman, A. (1994) Prospective randomised comparison of three surgical procedures for stress urinary incontinence: five year follow up. *Neurology and Urodynamics* **13**, 495–6

Hilton, P. and Mayne, C.J. (1991) The Stamey endoscopic bladder neck suspension: a clinical and urodynamic investigation, including actuarial follow-up over four years. *Br J Obstet Gynaecol* **98**, 1141–9

Marshall, V.F., Marchetti, A.A. and Krantz, K.E. (1949) The correction of stress incontinence by simple vesicourethral suspension. *Surg Gynecol Obstet* **88**, 509–18

Peattie, A. and Stanton, S.L. (1989) The Stamey operation for correction of genuine stress incontinence in the elderly woman. *Br J Obstet Gynaecol* **96**, 983–6

Pereyra, A.J. (1959) A simplified surgical procedure for the correction of stress urinary incontinence in women. *West J Surg Obstet Gynecol* **67**, 223–6

Pereyra, A.J. and Lebherz, T.B. (1967) The combined urethrovesical suspension and vaginourethroplasty for correction of urinary stress incontinence. *Obstet Gynecol* **30**, 537–46

Pereyra, A.J. and Lebherz, T.B. (1978) 'The revised Pereyra procedure' in H.J. Buchbaum and J.D. Schnidt (Eds) *Gynecologic and Obstetrical Urology* Chapter 13. Philadelphia: W.B. Saunders

Stamey, T.A. (1973) Endoscopic suspension of the vesical neck for urinary incontinence. *Surg Gynecol Obstet* **136**, 547–54

Stamey, T.A. (1980) Endoscopic suspension of the vesical neck for urinary incontinence in females. Report on 203 consecutive patients. *Ann Surg* **192**, 465–71

Further reading

Ashken, M.H., Abrams, P.H. and Lawrence, W.T. (1984) Stamey endoscopic bladder neck suspension for stress incontinence. *Br J Urol* **56**, 629–34

Hilton, P. (1989) A clinical and urodynamic study comparing the Stamey bladder neck suspension and suburethral sling procedures in the treatment of genuine stress incontinence. *Br J Obstet Gynaecol* **96**, 213

Lawrence, W.T. and Thomas, D.G. (1987) The Stamey bladder neck suspension operation for stress incontinence and neurovesical dysfunction. *Br J Urol* **59**, 305–10

Mundy, A.R. (1983) A trial comparing the Stamey bladder neck suspension procedure with colposuspension for the treatment of stress incontinence. *Br J Urol* **55**, 687

Raz, S. (1981) Modified bladder neck suspension for female stress incontinence. *Urology* **17**, 82

Stamey, T.A., Schaffer, A.J. and Condy, M. (1975) Clinical and roentgenographic evaluation of endoscopic suspension of the vesical neck for urinary incontinence. *Surg Gynecol Obstet* **140**, 355

11

Laparoscopic colposuspension

Jacqueline M. Lavin and A. R. B. Smith

Over the past 45 years, there have been two major developments in the management of stress incontinence. Firstly, the increasing use of pre-operative urodynamic assessment has led to a reduction in the number of patients with abnormal bladder function having inappropriate bladder neck surgery. Secondly, the abdominal/ retropubic approach has gained in popularity due to the ability to gain greater bladder neck elevation than would be possible vaginally, thereby producing higher success rates and a reduced risk of recurrence.

There have been many surgical techniques designed to cure stress incontinence. Unfortunately, the number of controlled studies with objective pre-operative and post-operative assessment, and with long-term follow-up is small. This makes comparison of the relative merits of the procedures difficult.

Most studies demonstrate that the abdominal/retropubic approach carries a higher success rate than vaginal surgery. However, increasing experience with retropubic surgery has led to the recognition that the higher cure rates are accompanied by an increased risk of post-operative voiding difficulty, detrusor instability, coital dysfunction and vaginal prolapse.

Minimally invasive techniques for colposuspension, such as described by Pereyra (1959) and Stamey (1973) have not produced results as good or long lasting as the conventional colposuspension first described by Burch in 1961. To date there are insufficient data to determine whether laparoscopic colposuspension represents an advance in the surgical management of stress incontinence in terms of cure and post-operative recovery or merely a further procedure in the long list of operations which have promised, but failed to produce a high cure rate with low morbidity. It is possible that the early return to normal activity associated with laparoscopic surgery will result in a higher incidence of recurrence, as has been the case with needle colposuspension. Well-controlled, randomised studies are required to evaluate the role of the laparoscopic approach.

Laparoscopic colposuspension

Excellent visualisation of the retropubic space can certainly be achieved with the laparoscope. However, the advantage of the shorter convalescence following laparoscopic colposuspension must be weighed against the capital cost of the equipment, the additional surgical expertise required and the risks inherent in laparoscopic surgery.

The first report on laparoscopic colposuspension by Vancaillie and Schuessler (1991) included 19 patients. Two of the first four patients required laparotomy to complete the procedure, indicating the technical difficulty of the operation. Lui (1992) reported a series of 58 patients with demonstrable primary stress incontinence and normal bladder function on simple cystometry. The intraperitoneal approach was employed and two Goretex sutures fixed the full thickness of the anterior vaginal wall to Cooper's ligament on each side. The cul-de-sac was obliterated with prolene sutures with a Moschowitz procedure (Moschowitz 1912). In this series of 58 patients, one sustained a bladder injury during surgery, which was repaired laparoscopically and another bled from the suprapubic catheter insertion. The suprapubic catheter was removed in all cases one week after surgery and no cases of voiding difficulty were reported. The patients were reviewed three months after surgery and none leaked with a standing stress test, although three patients had increased incontinence due to detrusor instability. The paper states that all patients were allowed to drive and return to work one week after surgery, provided their job did not require too much physical exertion.

Nezhat *et al.* (1994) performed a retrospective review of 62 women who underwent laparoscopic bladder neck surgery as a primary procedure. In 16 patients who either had or were thought likely to develop an enterocele, a Moschowitz procedure was employed. A single Ethibond suture was used in most cases to elevate the periurethral fascia to Cooper's ligament, or to the midline of the symphysis pubis cartilage 'depending on the surgeon's preference'. One intra-operative bladder injury occurred, which was repaired laparoscopically. Of the 62 cases, 58 were able to void on the second or third post-operative day. Post-operatively, five of the 62 had symptomatic leakage, of whom four had detrusor instability. No cases of vaginal prolapse were reported in this series.

A technique was developed by Presthus and Beadle (Ou *et al.* 1993), designed to overcome the difficulty of laparoscopic suturing. A prolene mesh was fixed to the para-urethral fascia and Cooper's ligament with a titanium stapler. The staples were applied through a disposable hernia stapling gun, the cost of which may be regained through reduced operating time. No case of failure was reported in a series of 40 patients with a mean of six months follow-up. There were no reported complications of staples in the anterior vaginal wall.

A further form of laparoscopic colposuspension has been described by Harewood (1993). In a series of seven patients a Stamey type of operation was performed under laparoscopic vision. Harewood suggests that the advantage of the laparoscopic approach is that it allows direct examination of the bladder and observation of the bladder neck during tying of the sutures. Despite this advantage, bladder perforation occurred in one case.

Burton (1994) published the only randomised control trial of laparoscopic and open colposuspension. In a series of 60 patients undergoing primary treatment for stress incontinence, full post-operative subjective and objective assessment was performed at six and 12 months. The procedure was performed through the peritoneal cavity and four polyglycolic acid sutures were placed in all cases. One bladder perforation occurred in each group. Subjectively, six out of the 30 women in the laparoscopic group leaked urine at 12 months compared with two out of the 30 in the open group. Although Burton performed ten laparoscopic colposuspensions prior to the study to familiarise himself with the technique, many authors would suggest more experience is advisable before conducting such a study.

The technique of laparoscopic colposuspension

Access is gained to the retropubic space by either the transperitoneal or the extraperitoneal approach.

In the transperitoneal approach, the peritoneal cavity is insufflated and the ports are inserted. In our unit, a 10 mm sub-umbilical port carries the laparoscope, with two further lateral ports, one 10 mm, for the scissors, sutures and pledget and the other 5 mm for the dissectors. Occasionally in the very obese, a central suprapubic port can help with tissue retraction. An intraperitoneal carbon dioxide pressure of 20 mmHg facilitates port insertion and haemostasis during the procedure.

The anterior abdominal wall peritoneum is opened using dissectors and scissors with monopolar diathermy above the level of the bladder and between the obliterated hypogastric artery folds. In obese patients these folds are less obvious, but in most patients there are vessels running in the lateral folds. If these vessels are not coagulated substantial haemorrhage may occur. The loose areolar connective tissue of the retropubic space can usually be divided easily with blunt dissection.

In the extraperitoneal approach, the retroperitoneal space is insufflated either directly, or by using a balloon device which is placed into the space and then inflated, exposing the retropubic space.

The bladder neck is then mobilised. A small pledget, held in tissue dissectors, is useful. It is advisable to secure a suture line to the pledget since, if it is dropped in the abdomen, it can be extremely difficult to find again. The bladder neck can then be mobilised by placing an index finger in the vagina and holding the dissector with the pledget in the other hand. As is the case with open colposuspension, mobilisation of the bladder neck is more difficult in patients who have had previous bladder neck surgery. Occasionally sharp dissection may be required. Venous bleeding may occur during the mobilisation and diathermy may be required. Haemorrhage is much less often found than with open procedures, partly because of the use of a pledget as opposed to a swab held by sponge forceps and partly due to the raised CO_2 pressure within the peritoneal cavity. We have not found the need to place a drain in the retropubic space at the end of the procedure. In the first 120 cases performed at St Mary's Hospital, Manchester, the only haematomas that we have encountered have been associated with the lateral port wounds.

Sutures are then placed in the para-urethral fascia and this is approximated to Cooper's ligament. We currently use PDS, since it is the strongest, most durable absorbable suture material available. We have found that suturing with a straight needle is generally much easier with two dimensional laparoscopic surgery. The orientation of a needle with a curve (either U-shaped or ski-shaped) can be extremely difficult in the retropubic space.

The predominant difference between open and laparoscopic colposuspension is the placement of sutures. In our unit, two sutures are placed on either side close together at the level of the proximal urethra when operating laparoscopically. At open colposuspension it is usual for a wider area of the fascia to be elevated with three sutures. However, when a vaginal examination is performed, it is not possible to detect this difference in suture placement. The sutures in the para-urethral fascia often perforate the full thickness of the vaginal wall and two bites are taken with each suture to reduce the risk of the suture tearing through the tissue.

A suprapubic catheter is then inserted, for two reasons. Firstly, when the colposuspension has been completed, the bladder is filled and this is a convenient method of checking that no bladder injury has occurred. Secondly, in our experience some patients experience a delay of more than seven days before spontaneous voiding can occur. A suprapubic catheter is more comfortable for the patient when voiding is delayed and repeated urethral catheterisation is avoided.

The anterior peritoneum may be closed, but this is not necessary if the peritoneal incision is large. A narrow gap in the peritoneum could lead to bowel entrapment. It is probable that in most cases re-peritonealisation occurs soon after the procedure.

There are increasing reports of laparoscopic port hernias. It would now seem prudent to close lateral ports wounds, particularly when more than 5 mm in diameter. Instruments are available to facilitate this.

Transperitoneal vs extraperitoneal

The transperitoneal approach allows other pelvic procedures to be performed including uterosacral ligament shortening and apposition, hysterectomy and sacrocolpopexy. It also offers a larger operating field.

The extraperitoneal route reduces the risk of bowel injury during port insertion and of bladder injury during opening of the peritoneum. This approach allows the lateral ports to be placed lower on the abdominal wall, which reduces the risk of injury to the inferior epigastric vessels and of hernia formation. Unfortunately, this also causes a reduction in the operating space available.

Hazards

Injury to the inferior epigastric vessels is a real concern to the laparoscopic pelvic surgeon. The lateral ports should be inserted under direct vision. Whilst careful insertion of the lateral ports will generally avoid injury, branches from these and other vessels may be injured and this may not be apparent during the procedure.

The risk of injury to the intra-abdominal viscera during open colposuspension is negligible, whilst placement of the ports into the peritoneal cavity during laparoscopic surgery will occasionally result in visceral injury which may not be recognised at the time of surgery. In a large series from France, one in 200 cases required laparotomy after laparoscopic surgery (Querleu *et al.* 1993).

There is a risk of injury to the fundus of the bladder on opening the peritoneum, particularly in those women who have undergone previous surgery, and in whom the bladder is elevated and dissection is more difficult on account of adhesions. This can best be avoided by dissection into the retropubic space lateral to the midline, since most adhesions from previous surgery occur centrally and are easier to identify when the space has been opened laterally.

Post-operative care

Analgesic requirements are variable, but generally much less than required for open colposuspension. Rectal diclofenac may avoid the need for narcotic analgesics.

We clamp the suprapubic catheter 36 hours after surgery and remove the suprapubic catheter when the residual urine is less than 150 ml. We have found that 60% of catheters can be removed by the fourth day, but voiding problems are not uncommon. In a series of 120 cases, long-term intermittent self-catheterisation has been necessary in one case.

At six-month follow-up, the results of our laparoscopic colposuspension appear comparable to those of patients who have undergone open colposuspension. In a group of primary and secondary procedures we have an 84% cure rate at six months.

Summary

As already stated, there is a need for careful evaluation of this technique. To date, the only prospective randomised controlled study of laparoscopic colposuspension is that carried out by Burton. However, prior to carrying out this trial he had only performed ten laparoscopic colposuspensions. We feel that the learning curve is longer than this. This is well illustrated by a 50% reduction in mean operating time noted over the first 50 cases in our series.

Colposuspension can be performed with laparoscopic assistance resulting in a faster return to normal life post-operatively. Only when five and 10-year follow-up have been performed will it be possible to evaluate whether this form of colposuspension is superior.

References

Burch, J.C. (1961) Urethrovaginal fixation to Cooper's ligament for correction of stress incontinence, cystocele and prolapse. *Am J Obstet Gynecol* **81**, 281–90

Burton, G. (1994) A randomised comparison of laparoscopic and open colposuspension. *Neurol Urodynamics* **13**, 497–8

Harewood, L.M. (1993) Laparoscopic needle colposuspension for genuine stress incontinence. *J Endourol* **7**, 319–22

Lui, C.Y. (1992) Laparoscopic retropubic colposuspension (Burch) procedure. *J Endourol* **6**, 137–41

Moschowitz, A.V. (1912) The pathogenesis, anatomy and cure of prolapse of the rectum. *Surg Gynecol Obstet* **15**, 7

Nezhat, C.H., Nezhat, F., Nezhat, C.R. and Rottenberg, H. (1994) Laparoscopic retropubic cystourethropexy. *J Am Assoc Gynecol Laparoscopy* **1**, 339–49

Ou, C.S., Presthus, J. and Beadle, E. (1993) Laparoscopic bladder neck suspension using hernia mesh and surgical staples. *J Laparoendosc Surg* **3**, 563–6

Pereyra, A.J. (1959) A simplified surgical procedure for the correction of stress urinary incontinence in women. *West J Surg Obstet Gynecol* **67**, 223–6

Querleu, D., Chapron, C., Chevallier, L. and Bruhat, M. (1993) Complications of gynecologic laparoscopic surgery – a French multicentre collaborative study. *N Engl J Med* **328**, 1355

Stamey, T.A. (1973) Endoscopic suspension of the vesical neck for urinary incontinence. *Surg Gynecol Obstet* **136**, 547–54

Vancaillie, T.G. and Schuessler, W. (1991) Laparoscopic bladder neck suspension. *J Laparoendosc Surg* **1**, 169–73

12

The fascial sling

Kristina Naidoo

Introduction

The concept of the bladder sling was originally described in 1907 by Giordano using gracilis muscle (Hohenfellner and Petri 1986). Later in Germany the placing of a fascial sling around the urethra was proposed (Stöeckel 1917; Goebell 1910).

In 1942 Aldridge described, in a single case report, the transplantation of strips of external oblique aponeurosis under the urethra for the relief of urinary stress incontinence. This method has since been widely adopted. Many other types of sling procedure have also been developed, varying in routes of access, type of material and sling tension.

Jeffcoate (1956) published the first series in the UK of patients who had undergone the Aldridge sling operation for stress incontinence. He reported 45 operations performed on women in whom he considered something more than anterior colporrhaphy was necessary, although his criteria were not defined. An 86% cure rate was obtained and Jeffcoate concluded that the value of this operation in properly selected cases is of a high order.

Indications

The sling procedure is primarily performed in patients who have undergone previous unsuccessful surgery for genuine stress incontinence. It is suitable when the urethra and paraurethral tissues are scarred and fibrotic or if the urethra is short and functionless.

It may be used as a primary procedure when there is vaginal narrowing or little bladder neck descent which would make anterior colporrhaphy or colposuspension technically difficult. Other indications include a low urethral closure pressure and previous pelvic radiation.

Operative technique

Numerous sling procedures and modifications have been described in the literature. Roseblade *et al.* (1993) in Manchester employed a technique very similar to that described by Aldridge in their series of 204 patients between 1980 and 1986. It is recounted here.

A low transverse abdominal incision is made and the rectus sheath divided in the line of the incision at least 4–5 cm above the symphysis. The fascia is reflected off the rectus muscles and these are separated in the midline to expose the retropubic space. The bladder neck is defined and dissected free on each side to accommodate the fascial sling.

Two 1 cm wide by 12 cm long strips of rectus sheath, external oblique fascia and occasionally some internal oblique fascia, depending on the condition of the tissues, are cut from the lower margin of the fascial incision and fashioned so that they hinge on one side about 2 cm from the midline. The free ends of the sling are detached as far as possible laterally and then passed in-between the rectus muscles into the retropubic space.

The dissection is completed vaginally through a longitudinal incision in the anterior vaginal wall. A 14 French Foley catheter helps to define the anatomy. The vaginal mucosa is reflected laterally off the proximal urethra and bladder neck. A tunnel is established by sharp and blunt dissection on either side of the bladder neck and the urogenital diaphragm opened to produce a communication between the retropubic space and vagina.

The free ends of the sling are brought down through the tunnel, placed around the bladder neck and secured to the pubocervical fascia without tension. A drain is left in the retropubic space and the rectus sheath closed with PDS (Ethicon, UK), a slowly absorbable suture. A suprapubic catheter is inserted and the urethral catheter removed. The operation is covered by prophylactic antibiotics.

The catheter remains on free drainage for five days after which it is clamped and the patient encouraged to void urethrally. The catheter clamp is only released for measuring residual urine volume or for the patient's comfort. Once the residual urine volume falls below 150 ml on two separate occasions the suprapubic catheter is removed.

This method can be modified if other sling materials are used. Jarvis and Fowlie (1985) used a porcine dermis sling, the central fusiform part of which was sutured underneath the bladder neck and the arms threaded up into the retropubic space, then sutured to the anterior rectus sheath. This requires a smaller abdominal incision than the rectus sheath sling.

Other techniques for the sling procedure include one where small lateral incisions in the rectus sheath are made with the retropubic space entered from below by dissection vaginally. A forceps is guided from the abdomen laterally to the bladder and urethra into the vagina where it grasps the sling material, withdrawing it to the abdominal incision on each side. The sling is fixed to the rectus fascia. Beck *et al.* (1988) used this technique with a fascia lata sling harvested from the patient's thigh. Other modifications include securing the sling to the ileo-pectineal ligament (Morgan *et al.* 1985).

A closed procedure without a vaginal incision (Chin and Stanton 1995) involves creating a suburethral tunnel through a lower abdominal incision, thus avoiding vaginal contamination. Other refinements include plication of the pubovesical fascia under the urethra which creates a strong base for the sling. Placement of a suburethral Martius fat-pad graft produces a base for the sling when the tissues are scarred, devascularised and fibrotic after previous surgery.

Bent (1990) advocated opening the bladder and endoscopy to ensure the bladder and ureters were intact and that the sling was placed in the correct location. Few surgeons would open a bladder for this reason, but some will routinely perform cystoscopy after the sling has been placed.

Sling materials

A wide variety of materials has been used for slings.

Organic sling material can be either autogenic, such as rectus sheath fascia (McGuire and Lytton 1978), fascia lata (Beck *et al.* 1988), palmaris longus (Poliak *et al.* 1984) and dermal graft (Pelosi *et al.* 1976), or allogenic, such as lyodura (Rottenberg *et al.* 1985) or porcine dermis (Jarvis and Fowlie 1985). Inorganic materials have also been used, such as plastic materials (Zoedler 1961), mersiline (Ridley 1966; Beck *et al.* 1974), Marlex mesh (Hilton and Stanton 1983; Morgan *et al.* 1985), silastic bonded Dacron (Chin and Stanton 1995) and Gore-tex® (Horbach *et al.* 1988).

Autogenic sling material needs to be harvested and may be of limited size and strength. Lyodura obtained from cadaverous dura mater may transmit Creutzfeldt-Jacob disease and should be used with caution. It is also very expensive. Porcine dermis is readily available, easy to handle, consistent in nature with a good tensile strength. In cases of infection the band dissolves, giving rise to no foreign body reaction as it is biologically immunologically inert (Iosif 1987).

Inorganic materials are non-absorbable and cause significant foreign body reaction. Slings of these materials are therefore prone to infection, rejection and erosion into the bladder or urethra with risks of fistula formation or even urethral transection.

Sling tension

There is no consensus regarding the degree of sling tension which should be applied. Appropriate tension is a difficult term to define and a common error is making the sling too tight.

Chin and Stanton (1995) using a silastic sling, Morgan *et al.* (1985) using Marlex mesh and Roseblade *et al.* (1993) with the rectus sheath fascial sling, all use minimal tension just sufficient to support the bladder neck and produce some elevation. Hodgkinson (1978) advocated moderate upward tension and Jarvis and Fowlie (1985) applied tension to a maximum achievable against a size 16 French urethral catheter.

Some surgeons have used intra-operative urethral pressure measurements to determine sling tension. McGuire and Lytton (1978) adjusted the sling tension so that there was an increase in urethral pressure of at least 10 cm of water in the region of the sling. Beck *et al.* (1988) created an intra-operative pressure of 80–90 cm of water at the sling site. Despite these measures, in their series of 170 patients there was a prolonged voiding interval of a mean of 59.6 days (range 13–270 days) from surgery to successful voiding. It seems that intra-operative pressure recordings do not sufficiently indicate how tight the sling will be post-operatively and cannot eliminate voiding problems.

Complications

Complications of the sling procedure include those associated with any major surgery, e.g. thromboembolism, as well as those specific to the procedure itself. Pre-operative counselling should include discussion about common complications as well as the chance of cure to allow the patient to make an informed decision about having surgery.

Intra-operative complications include haemorrhage during dissection of the retropubic space and vaginally. Trauma to the bladder and urethra necessitates formal closure. Fibrosis and distortion of normal anatomy following previous surgery make these complications more likely.

Early post-operative complications include pyrexia (incidence 15–80%) which may be due to either urinary tract infection (incidence 15–40%) and wound infection (incidence 5–30%). Prophylactic antibiotics, drainage of the retropubic space and suprapubic catheterisation avoiding repeated urethral catheterisation will reduce febrile morbidity.

The most troublesome long-term complications are voiding disorders with an incidence of 10.4% (range 2–20%) and de novo detrusor instability which occurs in 16.6% (4–29%) of cases (Jarvis 1994). Roseblade *et al.* (1993) in Manchester reported an incidence of voiding difficulty, defined as a residual urine of >100 ml at objective follow up at 6–12 months, as 7% (12 out of 174 patients). De novo detrusor instability was demonstrated at follow-up in six of 174 cases (3.5%).

Failure to establish voiding post-operatively or persistently high residual urine volumes may be managed by intermittent self catheterisation. Alternatively, a second procedure to decrease sling tension by stretching it, releasing it (McGuire and Lytton 1978) or removing it completely (Chin and Stanton 1995) can be performed.

A late complication with inorganic material is erosion into the urethra and bladder. Morgan *et al.* (1985) described two such cases of erosion into the urethra by marlex mesh. In both instances the sling was cut transurethrally with maintenance of continence in the short term.

Urinary fistulae have been reported. Chin and Stanton (1995) describe a vesico-vaginal fistula which occurred one month post-operatively. Successful vaginal repair was obtained and the sling did not need to be removed as it was not in the proximity of the fistula.

Incisional herniae of the abdominal scar following a rectus sheath fascial sling may occur.

Results

Published success rates for sling procedures vary considerably. Jarvis (1994) performed a review of all studies concerning surgical procedures for women with genuine stress incontinence from 1970 onwards. Prior to 1970 the concept of detrusor instability had not been fully recognised. Cure was defined as total continence of urine using an objective assessment, e.g. pad test, cystometry. The cure rate for the bladder sling as a first procedure was 93.9% and when performed for recurrent symptoms was 86.1%.

In the Manchester series of 204 patients (Roseblade *et al.* 1993) the fascial sling for genuine stress incontinence in the absence of detrusor instability produced continence in 151 of 174 patients (87%). This was assessed by repeat urodynamic studies 6–12 months after surgery.

Beck *et al.* (1988) reported that ten out of 13 sling failures redeveloped incontinence within six months of surgery. None of 17 patients followed for more than two years had recurrence of stress incontinence, suggesting the sling is capable of effective long-term cure. So far no long-term studies using objective measures have been reported so this impression has not been confirmed.

Cure rates are identical whether or not hysterectomy is performed (Stanton and Cardozo 1979). The outcome of surgery is not adversely affected by age, number of previous operations or low maximum urethral closure pressure (Roseblade *et al.* 1993).

Detrusor instability is not in itself a contraindication to sling procedure (McGuire and Lytton 1978). It will, however, reduce the cure rate. In the Manchester series (Roseblade *et al.* 1993) 30 patients also had detrusor instability prior to the fascial sling; surgery produced continence in 22 (73%) compared with 87% in the group with genuine stress incontinence alone. McGuire and Lytton (1978) reported an 80% cure in their group with genuine stress incontinence and motor urge incontinence. This increased to 91% when the detrusor instability was treated medically compared with a cure rate of 96% for genuine stress incontinence only.

Mechanism of action

The mechanism of action of the sling is not well understood. The principle of surgery is to provide posterior support to the bladder neck and sometimes bladder neck elevation. It has been postulated that any increase in intra-operative pressure will result in compression of the urethra against the sling, thereby increasing intra-urethral pressure (Stanton *et al.* 1985).

Conclusion

The bladder sling appears to produce a good cure rate with acceptable morbidity, particularly with an autogenic material. The incidence of voiding difficulty and de novo detrusor instability following surgery compares favourably with colposuspension.

References

Aldridge, A.H. (1942) Transplantation of fascia for relief of urinary stress incontinence. *Am J Obstet Gynecol* **44**, 398

Beck, R.P., Grove, D., Arnusch, D. and Harvey, J. (1974) Recurrent urinary stress incontinence treated by the fascia lata sling procedure. *Am J Obstet Gynecol* **120**, 613

Beck, R.P., McCormick, R.N. and Nordstrom, R.N. (1988) The fascia lata sling procedure for treating recurrent genuine stress incontinence of urine. *Obstet Gynecol* **72**, 699

Bent, A.E. (1990) Management of recurrent genuine stress incontinence. *Clin Obstet Gynecol* **33**, 358

Chin, Y.K. and Stanton, S.L. (1995) A follow up of silastic sling for genuine stress incontinence. *Br J Obstet Gynaecol* **102**, 143

Goebell, R. (1910) Operativen beseitigung der angeborenen. *Incontinentia Vesicae Z Gynäk Urol* **2**, 187

Hilton, P. and Stanton, S.L. (1983) Clinical and urodynamic evaluation of the polypropylene (Marlex) sling for genuine stress incontinence. *Neurourol Urodynam* **2**, 145–53

Hodgkinson, C.P. (1978) Recurrent stress urinary incontinence. *Am J Obstet Gynecol* **132**, 844

Hohenfellner, R. and Petri, E. (1986) 'Sling procedures' in S.L. Stanton and E.A. Tanagho (Eds) *Surgery of Female Incontinence* (2nd ed.) p. 106. London and Berlin: Springer Verlag

Horbach, N.S., Blanco, J.S., Ostergard, D.R. *et al.* (1988) A suburethral sling procedure with polytetrafluoroethylene for the treatment of genuine stress incontinence in patients with low urethral closure pressure. *Obstet Gynecol* **71**, 648–52

Iosif, S. (1987) Porcine corium sling in the treatment of urinary stress incontinence. *Arch Gynecol* **240**, 131

Jarvis, G.J. (1994) Surgery for genuine stress incontinence. *Br J Obstet Gynaecol* **101**, 371

Jarvis, G.J. and Fowlie, A. (1985) Clinical and urodynamic assessment of the porcine dermis bladder sling in the treatment of genuine stress incontinence. *Br J Obstet Gynaecol* **92**, 1189

Jeffcoate, T.N.A. (1956) The results of the Aldridge sling operation for stress incontinence. *J Urol* **119**, 82

McGuire, E.J. and Lytton, B. (1978) Pubo-vaginal sling procedure for stress incontinence. *J Urol* **119**, 82

Morgan, J.E., Farrow, G.A. and Stewart, F.E. (1985) The Marlex sling operation for the treatment of recurrent stress urinary incontinence: a 16 year review. *Am J Obstet Gynecol* **151**, 224

Pelosi, M.A., Langer, A., Sama, J.C. *et al.* (1976) Treatment of urinary stress incontinence. *Obstet Gynecol* **47**, 377

Poliak, A., Avrom, I. and Liebling, R.W. (1984) Sling operation for recurrent stress incontinence using the tendon of the palmaris longus. *Obstet Gynecol* **63**, 850–4

Ridley, J.H. (1966) Appraisal of the Goebell–Frangenhein–Stöeckel sling procedure. *Am J Obstet Gynecol* **95**, 74

Roseblade, C.K., Hosker, G.L., Smith, A.R.B. and Warrell, D.W. (1993) *Proceedings of the 23rd Annual Meeting ICS 93 Rome*, p. 127

Rottenberg, R.D., Weil, A., Brioschi, P.A. *et al.* (1985) Urodynamic and clinical assessment of the lyodura sling operation for urinary stress incontinence. *Br J Obstet Gynaecol* **92**, 829

Stöeckel, N. (1917) Uber die Verwendung der muculi pyradidale bei der operativen behandlung der. *Incontinentia Urinae Gynäk Urol* **41**, 11

Stanton, S.L., Brindley, G.S. and Holmes, D.M. (1985) Silastic sling for urethral sphincter incompetence in women. *Br J Obstet Gynaecol* **92**, 747

Stanton, S.L. and Cardozo, L.D. (1979) Results of the colposuspension operation for incontinence and prolapse. *Br J Obstet Gynaecol* **86**, 693

Zoedler, D. (1961) Zue operativen behandlung der weiblichen stress incontinenz. *Zentralbl Urol* **54**, 355

13

Management of failed continence surgery

Ash Monga and Stuart Stanton

Introduction

With the development of new surgical techniques and the high public expectation of success, we are increasingly aware of the need to discuss with patients beforehand the likely success and the complication rates of our treatment strategies. It is therefore important that we are aware of risk management and where the major risks of litigation lie. According to Department of Health statistics, clinical negligence claims are expected to increase by 25% per year. Litigation is no stranger to urinary incontinence, either because surgery has caused a previously continent patient to become wet or the continence procedure has failed.

A large number of operations have been designed to treat genuine stress incontinence (GSI or urethral sphincter incompetence). Whatever the procedure a proportion of patients will remain incontinent and a few may develop complications such as detrusor instability (DI), voiding difficulty or prolapse. Reported success rates for primary surgery often exceed 90% and for secondary surgery are invariably worse, with success rates approximately 7% lower (Jarvis 1994). There appears to be a time-dependent decline in success for ten years, after which it reaches a plateau (Alcalay *et al.* 1994). Identifying and comparing failure in the published literature is complicated by the following factors:

1 Studies comparing different surgical procedures do not use randomised patient selection criteria.
2 There is no standardisation of indications, inclusion or exclusion criteria.
3 There is a variation in surgical technique.
4 Many papers present surgical (clinical) data rather than objective data.
5 The definition of cure is imprecise and varies from one study to another, e.g. complete freedom from stress incontinence is not differentiated from relative improvement.
6 The length of follow-up is variable.

Aims of continence surgery

The aims of continence surgery are to:

1 Return the proximal urethra and bladder neck to a position where intra-abdominal pressure transmission to this region is identical to that transmitted to the bladder.

Table 13.1 Failure rates (%) of continence surgery

	Subjective	Objective	Detrusor instability	Voiding difficulty	Pain
Anterior repair	19	28	8	0	—
MMK	7	11	11	11–12	—
Colposuspension	10	16	10	12	12
EBNS	21	29	6	6–10	5
Sling	18	15	17	13	—
Injectable	44	40	—	—	—

(from Jarvis 1994).

2 Increase urethral resistance or pressure when it is below that of the intravesical pressure at rest.
3 Produce a combination of the above.
4 Repair any paravaginal fascial defects to restore anatomy (Shull 1989).
5 Restoration of the suburethral 'hammock support' (De Lancey 1991).

A variety of procedures exists but there is no consensus on the best operation; the chosen procedure should take into account clinical and urodynamic parameters. It is important to inform the patient of the objectives of the operation and its anticipated success rate and complications.

Definition of failure

Failure is defined as the recurrence of the symptom of stress incontinence or the occurrence of another type of incontinence. Most failures occur immediately or in the first post-operative year; some occur after this time and may be part of an ageing process or precipitated by increased physical activity. The following can occur:

1 The symptom of stress incontinence may persist due to inadequate surgical correction of genuine stress incontinence, or due to detrusor instability which may have been present preoperatively or is a *de novo* occurrence.
2 The symptom of urge incontinence may persist or occur *de novo.* This may be due to detrusor instability (DI).
3 A voiding disorder may result in retention with overflow, or the symptom of stress incontinence.
4 Continuous incontinence due to a fistula, either undetected preoperatively or secondary to the continence surgery.

Table 13.1 shows the failure rates of various continence procedures. In addition, the following complications may be encountered: urgency and frequency, voiding difficulty, prolapse and pain.

Definition of cure

Subjective measures should refer to cure of incontinence rather than improvement. Objective assessment of cure is the inability to demonstrate stress incontinence:

1 during clinical examination in both supine and standing positions;
2 on a 1-hour pad test, with a measured loss of less than 1 g;
3 by provocative cystometry or videocystourethrography;
4 by a positive distal urethral electrical conductance test;
5 during ambulatory monitoring.

The use of urethral pressure profilometry or ultrasound is not diagnostic.

Factors affecting outcome

1 Incorrect diagnosis of GSI
2 Choice of operation
3 Previous bladder neck surgery
4 Detrusor instability
5 Low pressure urethra
6 Denervation
7 Age and hysterectomy

Incorrect diagnosis of GSI

Failure to correctly diagnose genuine stress incontinence as the cause of stress incontinence may lead to continence surgery being used to treat a variety of causes of the symptom of stress incontinence, e.g. detrusor instability, overflow retention and urethral diverticulum.

Choice of operation

Failure may be related to incorrect choice of operation or a faulty technique. Traditionally most gynaecologists have performed an anterior repair as their first line continence procedure; however, a recent review of continence surgery shows that suprapubic operations are superior, although they are associated with increased complications (Jarvis 1994).

Suture material and patient activity

Longer lasting absorbable or permanent sutures have superseded catgut due to their maintained tensile strength. Suture breakage is rare, but is more likely to cause problems with needle suspension operations where success depends on a single suture either side of the bladder neck with little associated fibrosis and scarring. Sutures can tear through patient's tissues, as a result of sudden physical activity, which may happen more commonly in the elderly and patients with poorer quality connective tissue, e.g. on steroids.

Previous bladder neck surgery

Bladder neck surgery, whether intended to correct incontinence or anterior vaginal wall prolapse, is a well-documented risk factor for failure (Stanton *et al.* 1978; Hilton and Stanton 1983; Galloway *et al.* 1987; Hilton 1989), although some authors dispute this (Sand *et al.* 1987; Eriksen *et al.* 1990). At five-year follow-up, cure rates for primary surgery of 86% and secondary surgery of 67% are reported (Stanton *et al.* 1982). This difference persists at ten years with primary surgery objective cure rates of 81% and secondary surgery objective cure rates of 61% (Alcalay *et al.* 1994). Explanations vary: from technical difficulties encountered during secondary surgery, reduced vaginal mobility, periurethral fibrosis and scarring, to denervation and devascularisation resulting from dissection. Finally, the patient may have a congenital connective tissue weakness.

Detrusor instability

The presence of preoperative detrusor instability has been shown to have a deleterious effect on the outcome of continence surgery (Stanton *et al.* 1978; Pow-Sang *et al.* 1986). This appears to be accentuated in patients with systolic detrusor instability compared to low complaint detrusor instability (Wilkie *et al.* 1986), and the height of systolic contraction has an inverse relationship with success (Lockhart *et al.* 1984). However, McGuire (1985) and Blaivas and Oleson (1988) found the presence of preoperative detrusor instability to be of no predictive value although these statements were not confirmed by post-operative urodynamic studies.

Detrusor instability is a frequent post-operative problem, after colposuspension cumulative rates of 17% are reported (Vierhout and Mulder 1992), with lower rates ascribed to other procedures (Jarvis 1994). The cause of post-operative detrusor instability (DI) is unknown and unlike the male is not thought to be due to obstruction although this has been suggested (Brading and Turner 1994). A more likely explanation is the failure to detect preoperative DI by standard cystometry.

Low pressure urethra

Despite adequate elevation of the bladder neck during surgery, GSI persists in some patients presumably due to a decreased urethral resistance. McGuire (1981) reported a 41% failure rate if the maximum urethral closure pressure (MUCP) was less than $20\,cm\,H_2O$; Sand *et al.* (1987) described a group of 86 women undergoing colposuspension in whom patients with a preoperative MUCP less than $20\,cm\,H_2O$ were three times more likely to have an unsatisfactory outcome. The same group performed a case-controlled study with 21 patients in each group (Bowen *et al.* 1989). Of the successfully treated patients, 81% had an MUCP greater than $20\,cm\,H_2O$ compared to 23% of failures. These findings were confirmed by Wolf *et al.* (1989). In the latter study success rates fell from 91% to 75% if the MUCP was less than $20\,cm\,H_2O$ prior to colposuspension. An MUCP cut-off of $20\,cm\,H_2O$ also predicts the success of the Stamey procedure (Hilton, personal communication).

Whilst there is evidence that a low urethral pressure adversely influences surgical outcome, an absolute cut-off point remains unproven.

Denervation

Denervation attributed to childbirth has been documented both by electrophysiological tests and histologically (Snooks *et al.* 1986; Smith *et al.* 1989). Whether the extent of denervation affects the outcome of surgery has not been investigated.

Age and hysterectomy

An increased failure rate has been linked with increasing age (Stanton *et al.* 1978; Hilton 1989), especially if the MUCP is low (Meschia *et al.* 1993). This is thought to be associated with hypo-oestrogenism and consequent tissue atrophy, reduced vascularity and ineffective hermetic closure of the urethra. The association has been refuted (Eriksen *et al.* 1990).

The effect of concurrent hysterectomy at the time of colposuspension on outcome is disputed. Stanton *et al.* (1978) and Langer *et al.* (1988) reported no adverse influence; this is contested by Sand *et al.* (1988).

Adverse factors in failed colposuspension – retrospective study

Methods

In an ongoing analysis, clinical and urodynamic data have been retrieved from casenotes of 73 patients who have had a successful colposuspension and from 56 patients whose colposuspensions have failed. The effect of individual variables on success or failure has been analysed, using SPSS for PC.

Results

See Table 13.2.

Six patients had preoperative DI; four failed and two succeeded. Twelve patients complained of constipation; eight failed and four succeeded.

Hysterectomy performed prior to or at the time of colposuspension did not affect success of continence surgery. Preoperative posterior repair did not alter outcome.

Management of recurrent stress incontinence

The principles of management of recurrent stress incontinence are the same as those for primary surgery.

History and examination

The symptom of stress incontinence must be established as a significant complaint. Particular emphasis is placed on symptoms suggesting DI, neurological disease, fistula, voiding dysfunction or recurrent urinary tract infection, as these may complicate or contraindicate surgery.

Neurological and abdominal examination should be performed. Pelvic examination should assess residual urine, prolapse and uterine and adnexal pathology. The vaginal

Table 13.2   Analysis of variables on success or failure of colposuspension in 129 patients

Variable	Success	Failure	p
Mean age (years)	46 (32–70)	47 (23–67)	NS
Mean parity	2 (0–7)	3 (0–8)	p=0.077 NS
Heaviest infant (kg)	3.69 SD 0.7	3.63 SD 0.51	NS
Mean preop. weight (kg)	66 (49–84)	71 (53–99)	p<0.05
Absent urge and UI (n)	29	15	p=0.06 NS
Interrupt stream (n)	35	22	NS
Chronic cough (n)	9	7	NS
Primary (n)	55	34	
Secondary (n)	18	22	p<0.001

capacity and mobility are assessed to see whether the lateral vaginal fornices can be approximated to the pelvic side walls, to establish if a colposuspension is feasible. The vagina may be scarred and bladder neck mobility limited as a consequence of previous surgery.

Investigation

Urodynamic assessment is mandatory where further surgery is agreed. Oblique lateral videocystourethrography with uroflowmetry is the investigation of choice; if this is not available then cystometry is performed. The sign of stress incontinence requires confirmation, and detrusor instability and voiding problems should be identified. A pad test can be used to demonstrate loss and ambulatory monitoring may increase diagnostic sensitivity. The position and mobility of the bladder neck can be assessed. The use of urethral pressure profilometry has previously been discussed and remains controversial.

Choice of surgery

The patient's clinical and urodynamic characteristics must be matched with the characteristics of the surgery. Her clinical characteristics include frailty, position of bladder neck, vaginal scarring and any prolapse. The urodynamic features include position of bladder neck, urethral resistance, voiding difficulty and presence of detrusor instability. The features of the operation include success and morbidity, whether it elevates, obstructs or does both. If the bladder neck is not elevated then a colposuspension, Marshall Marchetti Krantz or endoscopic bladder neck suspension can be performed. If the bladder neck is already well elevated then the options include: (a) the sling operation which can be performed if the bladder neck is not

Table 13.3 Choice of continence surgery

	Elevate	*Both*	*Obstruct*
Vaginal	Anterior repair		Collagen
Suprapubic	MMK Paravaginal repair	Colposuspension Sling	AUS
Combined	EBNS e.g. Pereyra		

aligned with the symphysis in order to correct this; or (b) if there is a low pressure urethra, an obstructive procedure such as periurethral injection or implantation of an artificial urethral sphincter. When vaginal capacity or mobility is limited, especially in the nulliparous or elderly patient, an endoscopic suspension procedure may be chosen, as a colposuspension may not be technically feasible (see Table 13.3).

If detrusor instability is present, then surgery should be deferred until anticholinergics and bladder retraining have been tried. Technically, the exposure of the bladder neck, urethra and paravaginal fascia may be challenging because of scar tissue as a result of prior surgery.

Conclusions

When studies fail to agree, it is likely that a multifactorial cause is present. The appropriate operation should be carried out first after the diagnosis has been confirmed by urodynamic studies. The patient needs to be aware of the probability and types of failure. The role of connective tissue and degree of denervation on the outcome of surgery has yet to be evaluated.

References

Abrams, P., Blaivas, G., Stanton, S.L. *et al.* (1988) Standardisation of terminology of lower urinary tract function. *Scand J Urol Nephrol* (suppl.) **114**, 5–19

Alcalay, M., Monga, A.K. and Stanton, S.L. (1994) The Burch colposuspension – A 10–20 year follow up. *Br J Obstet Gynaecol* (submitted)

Blaivas, J. and Oleson, C. (1988) Stress incontinence: classification and surgical approach. *J Urol* **139**, 727–31

Bowen, L.W., Sand, P.K., Ostergard, D.R. and Franti, C.E. (1989) Unsuccessful Burch retropubic urethropexy. A case controlled urodynamic study. *Am J Obstet Gynecol* **160**, 452–8

Brading, A.F. and Turner, W.H. (1994) The unstable bladder: towards a common mechanism. *Br J Urol* **73**, 3–8

De Lancey, J.O.L. (1992) Three dimensional analysis of urethral support: the 'hammock' hypotheses'. *Neurourol Urodynam* **11**, 306–8

Eriksen, B.C., Hagen, B., Eik-Nes, S.H. *et al.* (1990) Long term effectiveness of the Burch colposuspension in female urinary stress incontinence. *Acta Obstet Gynecol Scand* **69**, 45–50

Galloway, N.I.M., Davies, N. and Stephenson, T.P. (1987) The complications of colposuspension. *Br J Urol* **60**, 122–4

Hilton, P. and Stanton, S.L. (1983) A clinical and urodynamic assessment of the Burch colposuspension for genuine stress incontinence. *Br J Obstet Gynaecol* **90**, 934–9

Hilton, P. (1989) A clinical and urodynamic study comparing the Stamey bladder neck suspension and suburethral sling procedures in the treatment of genuine stress incontinence. *Br J Obstet Gynaecol* **96**, 213–20

Jarvis, G.J. (1994) Surgery for genuine stress incontinence. *Br J Obstet Gynaecol* **101**, 371–4

Langer, R., Neuman, M., Ron-El, R. *et al.* (1989) The effect of total abdominal hysterectomy on bladder function in asymptomatic women. *Obstet Gynecol* **74**, 205–7

Lockhart, J., Vorstman, B. and Politano, V. (1984) Anti incontinence surgery in females with detrusor instability. *Neurourol Urodynam* **3**, 201–7

McGuire, E.J. (1981) Urodynamic findings in patients after failure of stress incontinence operations. *Prog Clin Biol Res* **78**, 351–60

McGuire, E.J. (1985) Abdominal procedures for stress incontinence. *Urol Clin North Am* **12**, 285–90

Meschia, M., Barbacini, P., Carena Maini, M. *et al.* (1991) Unsuccessful Burch colposuspension: analysis of risk factors. *Int Urogynecol J* **2**, 19–21

Pow-Sang, J., Lockhart, J., Suarez, A. *et al.* (1986) Female urinary incontinence: preoperative selection, surgical complications and results. *J Urol* **136**, 831–3

Sand, P.K., Bowen, L.W., Panganiban, R. and Ostergard, D.R. (1987) The low pressure urethra as a factor in failed retropubic urethropexy. *Obstet Gynecol* **69**, 399–402

Sand, P.K., Hill, R.C. and Ostergard, D.R. (1988) Incontinence history as a predictor of detrusor stability. *Obstet Gynecol* **71**, 257–60

Shull, B.L. and Baden, W.F. (1989) A six year experience with paravaginal defect repair for stress urinary incontinence. *Am J Obstet Gynecol* **160**, 1432–40

Smith, A.R.B., Hosker, G.L. and Warrell, D.W. (1989) The role of partial denervation of the pelvic floor in the aetiology of genitourinary prolapse and stress incontinence of urine. A neurophysiological study. *Br J Obstet Gynaecol* **96**, 29–32

Snooks, S.J., Swash, M., Setchell, M. and Henry, M.M. (1986) Injury to the innervation of the pelvic floor sphincter musculature. *Lancet* **ii**, 546–50

Stanton, S.L., Cardozo, L.D., Williams, J. *et al.* (1978) Clinical and urodynamic features of failed incontinence surgery in the female. *Obstet Gynecol* **51**, 515–20

Stanton, S.L., Hertogs, K., Cox, C. *et al.* (1982) Colposuspension for genuine stress incontinence: a five year study. *Proceedings of the 12th Annual Meeting of the International Continence Society*, Leiden, Netherlands, pp. 618–20

Stanton, S.L. (1990) 'Why operations fail' in J.O. Drife, P. Hilton and S.L. Stanton (Eds) *Micturition. Proceedings of the 21st RCOG Study Group*, pp. 247–67. London: Springer-Verlag

Vierhout, M.E. and Mulder, A.F.P. (1992) De novo detrusor instability after Burch colposuspension. *Acta Obstet Gynecol Scand* **71**, 414–16

Wilkie, D., Barzilai, M. and Stanton, S.L. (1986) Combined urethral sphincter incompetence and detrusor instability: does colposuspension help? *Proceedings of the 16th Annual Meeting of the International Continence Society*, Boston, pp. 618–20

Wolf, H., Coburg, P. and Maass, H. (1989) Recidivrate nach intontinenzoperationen bei patrentinnen mit hypotoner urethra. *Geburtshilfe und Frauenheilkunde* **49**, 865–71

14

Detrusor instability – drugs and behavioural therapies

Linda Cardozo and Vik Khullar

Introduction

Detrusor instability is the second most common cause of urinary incontinence in women and accounts for 30–50% of cases (Torrens and Griffiths 1974). Genuine stress incontinence is the most common cause of urinary incontinence in premenopausal women but the incidence of detrusor instability is higher in the elderly and increases with increasing age. 'Idiopathic' detrusor instability has been considered as a variant of normal, being diagnosed in asymptomatic continent women on laboratory and ambulatory urodynamics (Robertson *et al.* 1994).

Aetiology

The bladder in the neonate contracts at a specific volume and control is learnt in infancy during 'potty training'. An unstable bladder may occur because of a failure to learn this control or because it reverts to its pre-trained state. In most women no cause can be found although possibly in some cases detrusor instability may be psychosomatic in origin. Increased neurosis has been found in women with detrusor instability (Norton *et al.* 1990) but the severity of the psychoneuroticism has a strong association with increasing incontinence symptoms (Moore *et al.* 1992), and reduced quality of life (Kelleher *et al.* 1993a). Neurological lesions such as multiple sclerosis and spinal injuries may cause uninhibited detrusor contractions, but this is only in a small number of women. In these women the bladder dysfunction is described as detrusor hyper-reflexia. Following incontinence surgery women have an increased incidence of detrusor instability (Cardozo *et al.* 1979). There is no specific cause; however, extensive dissection around the bladder neck may be a factor as it is more common after multiple previous operations; alternatively, the diagnosis of detrusor instability may be missed prior to surgery. Outflow obstruction is rare in women and does not seem to produce detrusor instability as seen with men suffering from prostatic hypertrophy. In the elderly the increased incidence of detrusor instability may be due to occult neuropathy, e.g. senile atherosclerosis or dementia.

Symptoms

The most common symptoms are urgency and frequency (Cardozo and Stanton 1980; Larsson *et al.* 1991), but there are many other causes for these symptoms so they are not diagnostic. Frequency develops as a result of the woman's attempt to reduce urinary leakage by regularly emptying her bladder. Nocturia is a common symptom in detrusor instability occurring in 70% of cases (Cardozo and Stanton 1980). Nocturia increases with age; over the age of 70 years it is normal to void twice at night and three times over the age of 80 years.

Urge incontinence is urinary leakage preceded by a strong desire to void, usually due to an involuntary detrusor contraction. Some women do not get this sensation and may only notice that they are wet. Leakage during sexual intercourse occurs in 35% of women with detrusor instability; 80% of women with detrusor instability suffer from sexual dysfunction (Kelleher et al. 1993b). Urinary incontinence at orgasm is more likely to occur in women with detrusor instability whereas those who leak on penetration usually have genuine stress incontinence. There appears to be a strong link between nocturnal enuresis and idiopathic detrusor instability.

On clinical examination it is important to note any urinary leakage, excoriation or a damp perineum. Alteration in sensation in the 'saddle area' of the perineum supplied by sacral roots S_2, S_3 and S_4 is found if a neurological lesion is present.

Investigations

A mid-stream specimen of urine should be sent for culture and sensitivity in all cases of urinary incontinence. A urinary tract infection can produce spurious urinary symptoms and misleading results from urodynamic tests.

A frequency/volume chart or urinary diary is a useful method of evaluating the woman's fluid intake and voided volumes. All parameters measured overlap with the measurements obtained from frequency/volume charts of women suffering from genuine stress incontinence (Larsson and Victor 1992). Uroflowmetry in idiopathic detrusor instability shows a high flow rate of short duration with a small voided volume. The measurement of the peak flow rate and the post-micturition urinary residual are important as these measures determine whether the woman is suffering from voiding difficulties with a large urinary residual. These women may also present with urgency and frequency of micturition.

Detrusor instability can be diagnosed during the filling and phase of the cystometrogram in about 50% of cases. The International Continence Society defines this as any uninhibited detrusor pressure rise associated with the symptom of urgency. There are different types of pressure rise: systolic detrusor contractions during filling, or detrusor contractions provoked by coughs, or detrusor contractions on standing. During filling a tonic pressure rise (low compliance) may be seen; this can be due to active contraction of the detrusor (in detrusor instability), passive stretching of the bladder wall (fibrosis of the bladder wall), or pressure from a pelvic mass (fibroid uterus) and may be difficult to differentiate from systolic detrusor contractions. In low compliance due to detrusor instability, the detrusor pressure falls exponentially when bladder filling is stopped. This is due to the active contraction of the detrusor relaxing after filling and does not occur with the other causes of low compliance. Both systolic detrusor instability and conditions causing low compliance produce the symptoms of urgency and frequency. During cystometry the patient should be questioned about symptoms and these should be related to the changes on the cystometrogram, in particular if the woman complains of marked urgency associated with detrusor contractions. Other features seen during urodynamics are small initial voided volume, early first sensation, small bladder capacity. During voiding the patient can experience difficulty in interrupting her urinary stream and a high isometric detrusor contraction may be seen. On videocystourethrography where contrast is used to fill the bladder, trabeculation of the bladder may be seen and prolonged milkback of contrast from the urethra back to the bladder after voiding is interrupted. Vesicoureteric reflux may also be seen especially in women with detrusor hyper-reflexia.

Cystourethroscopy is useful to exclude calculi and tumours and if a patient is resistant to pharmacological treatment. A biopsy can be taken to exclude interstitial cystitis. The bladder in women with long-standing detrusor instability is often trabeculated.

Treatment

General advice

Advice should be given on simple measures such as limiting drinking to less than 1.5 litres a day and to avoid tea, coffee, alcohol and any other beverages which may exacerbate their urinary problem (Griffiths *et al.* 1993). Other drugs such as diuretics, or gastrointestinal motility stimulants (cisapride) should be changed for other options (Gormley *et al.* 1993). If urinary leakage only occurs in specific situations such as during aerobics then a tampon inserted into the vagina may help maintain continence but this is of more use in women with genuine stress incontinence. The use of hormone replacement therapy to treat symptoms of urgency, frequency and nocturia may help in increasing the sensory threshold of the bladder but does not appear to cure detrusor instability (Fantl *et al.* 1994).

Drugs

Drugs to treat detrusor instability can be grouped into three broad categories according to their mode of action. They can reduce bladder contractility, increase outflow resistance or reduce urine production. Drugs reducing bladder contractility are classified as anticholinergics, antispasmodics or spasmolytics, tricyclic antidepressants, calcium channel blockers and prostaglandin synthetase inhibitors.

Anticholinergic drugs

These drugs produce competitive blockade of acetylcholine receptors at postganglionic parasympathetic receptors. Anticholinergic drugs are not specific for the bladder and produce antimuscarinic activity in many organ systems. As the drugs have similar mechanisms of action the side-effects produced are similar. The typical side-effects experienced by patients are a dry mouth due to suppression of salivary and oropharyngeal secretions, constipation due to reduced gastrointestinal motility, an increase in heart rate due to vagal blockade, and transient blurring of vision from blockade of the sphincter of the iris and the ciliary muscle of the lens of the eye. Dry mouth is the commonest symptom; the others are more likely to occur with increasing doses.

Anticholinergic drugs should not be used in patients with cardiac arrhythmias or those suffering from narrow-angle glaucoma. Propantheline bromide is a quaternary ammonium compound used at doses of 15–30 mg qds, but often higher doses are required. There are side-effects but it has been found to reduce bladder contractions (Holmes *et al.* 1989). A double-blind placebo-controlled cross-over trial of propantheline (15 mg tds and 60 mg nocte) in 20 incontinent women showed a significant decrease in nocturnal enuresis while the patients took propantheline (Whitehead 1967). The drug may be incompletely absorbed if the stomach is full.

Emepronium carageenate has superseded emepronium bromide because the latter caused oral and oesophageal ulceration. Using emepronium carageenate in a dose titration trial using oral doses 1200 mg, 1600 mg, 2000 mg per day in 72 women with detrusor instability, there was an improvement in symptoms without serious side-effects; this was corroborated by improved urodynamic findings (Massey and Abrams 1986). It must be stressed that this was not a double-blind placebo-controlled study so we must be cautious in our interpretation of the results. This drug is not available in the United Kingdom.

Spasmolytic drugs

Oxybutynin chloride is a tertiary amine compound with strong musculotrophic antispasmodic and local anaesthetic effects. It also has some anticholinergic and antihistaminic properties. Oxybutynin has been shown to be effective in both neuropathic (Thompson *et al.* 1976; Hehir *er al.* 1985; Gajewski and Awad 1986) and non-neuropathic (Moisey *et al.* 1980; Holmes *et al.* 1989; Tapp *et al.* 1990) bladder dysfunction. Intravesical instillation of oxybutynin has recently been shown to be efficacious in the treatment of severe detrusor instability and detrusor hyper-reflexia without the problem of distressing systemic anticholinergic side-effects (Madersbacher *et al.* 1991). The drug appears to be well absorbed from the bladder, and compared to oral intake the resorption is protracted with lower and later peak serum levels.

There have been a number of double-blind placebo-controlled trials (Thompson *et al.* 1976; Moisey *et al.* 1980; Riva and Casolati 1984; Cardozo *et al.* 1987); all have shown symptomatic as well as cystometric improvements with oxybutynin. The greatest problem has been compliance in taking the drug and the anticholinergic side-effects. This has been the reason why 10–23% of women discontinue oxybutynin (Gajewski and Awad 1986; Kirkali and Whitaker 1987; Baigre *et al.* 1988). Compliance has been improved through the use of lower doses, 2.5 mg and 3 mg bd, and gradually increasing the dose from a low starting level (Moore *et al.* 1990). Oxybutynin is one of the most useful drugs in the treatment of detrusor instability but the side-effects limit the drug's usefulness and it must be given frequently.

Flavoxate hydrochloride is a muscle relaxant with analgesic and local anaesthetic actions. The majority of studies have compared flavoxate with other drugs including flavoxate 200 mg qds compared with propantheline 30 mg qds. In 20 patients there were no significant differences between the two groups (Pedersen 1977). In comparison with emepronium bromide 200 mg tds in 38 patients, flavoxate relieved frequency and urgency and produced a greater increase in bladder capacity. In a four-week, double-blind cross-over study comparing a combination of flavoxate hydrochloride and emepronium bromide with placebo in the treatment of detrusor instability in 20 elderly women there were pharmacological effects but there was no effect on the women clinically. Thus flavoxate is not considered to be effective in detrusor instability.

Tricyclic antidepressants

Tricyclic antidepressants, particularly imipramine (Tofranil) are effective both in the facilitation of urine storage and increasing bladder outlet resistance. Imipramine has at least three modes of action, namely: central and peripheral anticholinergic effects; blockage of the active presynaptic re-uptake of the amine neurotransmitters noradrenaline and serotonin; and a sedative action probably related to antihistamine properties. It also appears to have a strong direct inhibitory effect on the detrusor smooth muscle which is neither cholinergic nor adrenergic and is possibly related to a local anaesthetic action. Additionally the effects of imipramine on the lower urinary tract appear to be additive to those of other anticholinergic drugs (Wein 1990). Castleden *et al.* (1981) have shown that a single night-time dose up to 150 mg of imipramine is effective in the treatment of detrusor instability in the elderly.

Imipramine is particularly indicated in the treatment of detrusor instability associated with predominantly nocturnal symptoms, coital incontinence, and in patients with mixed detrusor instability and urethral sphincter incompetence. Care must be exercised in the use of this drug in the elderly where postural hypotension and myocardial depressant effects can be a problem (Glassman *et al.* 1981), and the use of imipramine is contraindicated in patients receiving mono-amine-oxidase inhibitors.

Calcium channel blockers

Calcium ions are required for the excitation and contraction of bladder smooth muscle. Subjective and objective improvement have been found in patients taking nifedipine, an antihypertensive and antianginal drug; there is a reduction in the size and frequency of unstable contractions and increase in bladder capacity (Forman *et al.* 1978; Rud *et al.* 1979). Intravesical verapamil during cystometry has a similar effect on neuropathic bladders (Mattiasson *et al.* 1987). More studies are required on this class of drugs to determine their efficacy compared with other drugs used on the bladder. Terodiline hydrochloride, a drug with calcium channel blocking and antimuscarinic activity was very successful in the treatment of detrusor instability, but was voluntarily withdrawn after deaths due to cardiac arrhythmias.

DDAVP (Desmopressin)

DDAVP (1-Deamino, 8-Arginine Vasopressin), an analogue of Anti Diuretic Hormone (ADH), is used for women with intractable nocturia, or nocturnal enuresis. It is administered intra-nasally at bed-time (as either a spray or snuff), and is known to reduce nocturnal urine production by up to 50% (Hilton and Stanton 1982). It can, however, only be used once in a twenty-four hour period and results in a subsequent diuresis. An oral preparation of this drug is now available. Caution must

Table 14.1   A regime for bladder drill

1   Exclude underlying pathology.
2   Explain rationale of the regime to the patient.
3   Instruct the patient to void strictly by the clock (a suitable starting interval is one hour).
4   When the patient is dry and comfortable with the one-hour interval, it should be increased by 30-minute increments up to an interval of three hours.
5   A normal fluid intake should be maintained (1.5 hours).
6   A strict fluid balance chart must be maintained by the patient.
7   Encouragement and motivation are an important part of the regime.

(from Jarvis 1980)

be exercised in the use of DDAVP in the elderly, where fluid retention and cardiac compromise can be a serious problem (Carter *et al.* 1992). Evidence suggests that it is safe for use in the long term (Rew and Rundle 1989).

Behavioural treatment

There are many behavioural intervention studies attempting to treat urgency and frequency in women. Unfortunately, a significant proportion do not have a urodynamic diagnosis of detrusor instability as one of the entry criteria. Thus the groups of women studied are not homogeneous and the conclusions not necessarily valid for detrusor instability.

The success of behavioural intervention in the treatment of detrusor instability relies on the re-establishment of cortical control over the uninhibited bladder. Thus the normal pattern of regular voiding is regained. The bladder escaping the inhibition of the higher centres of the brain is supported by the provocation of sensory stimuli such as running water, putting a key in a lock, stress or anxiety produce urgency and urinary incontinence.

A number of authors have described a strong association between psychological disorders and the symptoms of urgency, frequency and urge incontinence (Frewin 1984; Freeman *et al.* 1985; Macauley *et al.* 1987). Moore (1989) found that women with lower psychoneurotic scores on the Crown Crisp Experiential Index responded better to treatment with oxybutynin than women with more abnormal psychoneurotic results. However, Morrison and colleagues (1986) studied 226 women undergoing investigation for urinary incontinence using the Eysenck Personality Inventory and found a relationship between incontinence and neuroticism, but no specific link between detrusor instability and neuroticism. Walters *et al.* (1990) and Moore *et al.* (1992) more recently found that neuroticism correlated well with the severity of urinary incontinence; the worse the urinary incontinence the greater the psychoneuroticism. This emphasises the effect that urinary incontinence has on women, not only to their lives, but their mental wellbeing.

Bladder drill

Bladder drill attempts to achieve continence by re-establishing cortical control of the unstable bladder. The women are instructed to empty their bladders at regular intervals, whether they have an urge to void or not (see Table 14.1). It is important that voiding is not attempted between these times and the time between each timed void is gradually increased over a number of days. This simple technique requires rigid adherence by the patient for success. A frequency/volume chart is used to record the times of micturition and volumes voided. As the bladder is retrained, the reinstated voluntary control dictates the pattern of voiding, not the unstable contractions.

Frewen was the first to report the results of bladder drill. The patients in his initial two studies did not have urodynamic studies (Frewen 1970, 1972). Subsequently a series of 40 patients with detrusor instability was found to achieve symptomatic and objective cure in 83% after three months (Frewen 1978). Symptomatic cure was found to precede the return to normal cystometry in this series. This level of symptomatic cure has been repeated by other groups (Fantl *et al.* 1981; Jarvis 1981). The long-term cure was impressive with 86% at six year follow-up (Frewen 1984) and 50% three years after treatment (Holmes *et al.* 1983). The later study included patients with the 'urge syndrome'; the initial cure rate was 85% but there was a 43% relapse rate.

A placebo-controlled study carried out by Jarvis (1982) involved 60 women who were allocated to inpatient bladder drill or an untreated control group after cystoscopy under general anaesthesia and cystometry. After three months 90% of the bladder drill group were continent and 83% were symptom-free compared with 23% in the control group.

Bladder drill appears to be an effective method of treating detrusor instability. The response rate is determined by patient compliance with the treatment regimen (Oldenburg and Millard 1986). This is influenced by enthusiastic patient contact, reassurance, long-term support and follow-up. Success is also improved if bladder drill is carried out as an inpatient procedure but this is expensive and prevents its wider use. Bladder drill should be first-line treatment for detrusor instability because the success rate is good, and the costs involved minimal if carried out on an outpatient basis (Fantl *et al.* 1991).

Other forms of behavioural therapy include psychotherapy, hypnotherapy (Freeman and Baxby 1982), and biofeedback (Cardozo *et al.* 1978). Biofeedback is of particular value in children (Van Gool *et al.* 1989) and uses modified urodynamic equipment to provide an auditory or visual signal to the patient about unstable detrusor contractions which they attempt to inhibit. These treatments are very labour intensive and confer little additional benefit over conventional bladder drill.

Acupuncture

There are several mechanisms of action of acupuncture on the bladder, none of which has yet been substantiated. Acupuncture has widespread effects on endogenous opioids and on the autonomic nervous system which may be of relevance (Murray *et al.* 1982). A number of studies have demonstrated the efficacy of acupuncture in the management of nocturnal enuresis (Song Baozhu 1985; Bartocci and Lucentini 1981). Philp *et al.* (1988) found a 76% symptomatic cure in patients with idiopathic detrusor instability and predominantly daytime symptoms, and a recent study using minimal stimulation acupuncture has shown it to be as effective as conventional anticholinergic therapy in the management of irritative bladder symptoms (Kelleher *et al.* 1994).

Conclusion

Detrusor instability affects many women and produces adverse symptoms. It causes embarrassment and can significantly impair the quality of life. There are different treatments for detrusor instability, none of which is wholly satisfactory. This is due to our lack of understanding of the aetiology of detrusor instability. Bladder training is a useful first-line therapy as the detrusor instability may be cured with minimal side-effects. The majority of women are treated with drugs which they may need to take indefinitely, as the symptoms return on stopping the medication. Current treatments may not cure the condition but distressing symptoms can be ameliorated and in this way improve the woman's quality of life.

References

Baigre, R.J., Kelleher, J.P., Fawsett, D.P. *et al.* (1988) Oxybutynin: Is it safe? *Br J Urol* **62**, 319–21

Bartocci, C. and Lucentini, M. (1981) Acupuncture and micromassage in the treatment of idiopathic night enuresis. *Minerva Med* **72**, 2235–6

Cardozo, L.D. and Stanton, S.L. (1980) Genuine stress incontinence and detrusor instability: a review of 200 cases. *Br J Obstet Gynaecol* **87**, 184–90

Cardozo, L.D., Abrams, P., Stanton, S.L. *et al.* (1978) Idiopathic bladder instability treated by biofeedback. *Br J Urol* **50**, 521–3

Cardozo, L.D., Stanton, S.L. and Williams, J.E. (1979) Detrusor instability following surgery for genuine stress incontinence. *Br J Urol* **51**, 204–7

Cardozo, L.D., Cooper, D. and Versi, E. (1987) Oxybutynin chloride in the management of idiopathic detrusor instability. *Neurourol Urodyn* **6**, 256–7

Carter, P.G., McConnell, A.A. and Abrams, P. (1992) The safety and efficacy of DDAVP in the elderly. *Neurourol Urodyn* **11**, 421–2

Castelden, C.M., George, C.F. and Benwick, A.J. (1981) Imipramine: a possible alternative to current therapy for urinary incontinence in the elderly. *J Urol* **125**, 318–20

Fantl, J.A., Hurt, W.G. and Dunn, L.J. (1981) Detrusor instability syndrome: the use of bladder retraining drills with and without anticholinergics. *Am J Obstet Gynecol* **140**, 885–8

Fantl, J.A., Wyman, J.F., McClish, D.K. *et al.* (1991) Efficacy of bladder training in older women with urinary incontinence. *JAMA* **265**, 609–13

Fantl, J.A., Cardozo, L.D. and McClish, D.K. (1994) Estrogen therapy in the management of urinary incontinence in postmenopausal women: a meta-analysis. First report of the hormones and urogenital therapy committee. *Obstet Gynecol* **83**, 12–18

Forman, A., Andersson, K.E., Henriksson, L. *et al.* (1978) Effects of nifedipine on the smooth muscle of the human urinary bladder in vitro and in vivo. *Acta Pharmacol Toxicol* **43**, 111–18

Freeman, R.M. and Baxby, K. (1982) Hypnotherapy for incontinence caused by the unstable bladder. *BMJ* **284**, 1831–4

Freeman, R.M., McPherson, F.M. and Baxby, K. (1985) Psychological features of women with idiopathic detrusor instability. *Urol Int* **40**, 247–59

Frewen, W.K. (1970) Urge and stress incontinence: fact and fiction. *Br J Obstet Gynaecol* **77**, 932–5

Frewen, W.K. (1972) Urgency incontinence: review of 100 cases. *Br J Obstet Gynaecol* **79**, 77–9

Frewen, W.K. (1978) An objective assessment of the unstable bladder of psychosomatic origin. *Br J Urol* **50**, 246–9

Frewen, W.K. (1984) The significance of the psychosomatic factor in urge incontinence. *Br J Urol* **56**, 330–2

Gajewski, J.B. and Awad, S.A. (1986) Oxybutynin versus propantheline in patients with multiple sclerosis and detrusor hyperreflexia. *J Urol* **135**, 966–9.

Glassman, A.H. and Bigger, J.T. (1981) Cardiovascular effects of therapeutic doses of tricyclic antidepressants: a review. *Arch Gen Psychiatr* **38**, 815–19

Gormley, E.A., Griffiths, D.J., McCracken, P.N. and Harrison, G.M. (1993) Polypharmacy and its effect on urinary incontinence in a geriatric population. *Br J Urol* **71**, 265–9

Griffiths, D.J., McCracken, P.N., Harrison, G.M. and Gormley, E.A. (1993) Relationship of fluid intake to voluntary micturition and urinary incontinence in geriatric patients. *Neurourol Urodyn* **12**, 1–7

Hehir, M. and Fitzpatrick, J.M. (1985) Oxybutynin and the prevention of urinary incontinence in spina bifida. *Eur Urol* **11**, 254–6

Hilton, P. and Stanton, S.L. (1982) The use of desmopressin (DDAVP) in nocturnal urine frequency in the female. *Br J Urol* **54**, 252–5

Holmes, D.M., Montz, F.J. and Stanton, S.L. (1989) Oxybutynin versus propantheline in the management of detrusor instability. A patient-regulated variable dose trial. *Br J Obstet Gynaecol* **96**, 607–12

Holmes, D.M., Stone, A.R., Bary, P.R. *et al.* (1983) Bladder training – three years on. *Br J Urol* **55**, 660–4

Jarvis, G.J. (1981) A controlled trial of bladder drill and drug therapy in the management of detrusor instability. *Br J Urol* **53**, 565–8

Jarvis, G.J. (1982) Bladder drill for the treatment of enuresis in adults. *Br J Urol* **55**, 178–80

Kelleher, C.J., Khullar, V. and Cardozo, L.D. (1993a) Psychoneuroticism and quality of life impairment in healthy incontinent women. *Neurourol Urodyn* **12**, 393–4

Kelleher, C.J., Cardozo, L.D., Khullar, V. *et al.* (1993b) The impact of urinary incontinence on sexual function. *J Sexual Health* **8**, 186–91

Kelleher, C.J., Filshie, J., Khullar, V. and Cardozo, L.D. (1994) Acupuncture in the treatment of irritative bladder symptoms. *J Br Med Acupunc Soc* (in press)

Kirkali, Z. and Whitaker, R.H. (1987) The use of oxybutynin in urologic practice. *Int Urol Nephrol* **19**, 385–91

Larsson, G., Abrams, P. and Victor, A. (1991) The frequency/volume chart in detrusor instability. *Neurourol Urodyn* **10**, 533–43

Larsson, G. and Victor, A. (1992) The frequency/volume chart in genuine stress incontinent women. *Neurourol Urodyn* **11**, 23–31

Macaulay, A.J., Stern, R.S., Holmes, D.M. *et al.* (1987) Micturition and the mind: psychological factors in the aetiology and treatment of urinary symptoms in women. *BMJ* **294**, 540–3

Madersbacher, H., Knoll, M. and Kiss, G. (1991) Intravesical application of oxybutynin: mode of action in controlling detrusor hyperreflexia. *Neurourol Urodyn* **10**, 375–6

Massey, J.A. and Abrams, P. (1986) Dose titration in clinical trials. An example using emepronium carrageenate in detrusor instability. *Br J Urol* **58**, 125–8

Mattiasson, A., Ekstrom, B. and Andersson, K.E. (1987) Effects of intravesical instillation of verapamil in patients with detrusor hyperactivity. *Neurourol Urodyn* **6**, 253–5

Moisey, C.V., Stephenson, T.P. and Brendler, C.B. (1980) The urodynamic and subjective results of treatment of detrusor instability with oxybutynin chloride. *Br J Urol* **52**, 472–5

Moore, K.H., Eadie, A.S., McAlister, A. *et al.* (1989) Response to drug treatment of detrusor instability in relation to psychosomatic. *Neurourol Urodyn* **8**, 412–13

Moore, K.H., Hay, D.M., Imrie, A.H. *et al.* (1990) Oxybutynin chloride (3 mg) in the treatment of women with idiopathic detrusor instability. *Br J Urol* **66**, 479–85

Moore, K.H., Richmond, D.H., Sutherst, J.R. and Manasse, P. (1992) Is severe 'wetness' associated with severe 'madness' in detrusor instability? *Neurourol Urodyn* **11**, 460–1

Morrison, L.M., Eadie, A.S., McAlister, A. *et al.* (1986) Personality traits in 226 patients with urinary incontinence. *Br J Urol* **58**, 387–9

Murray, K.H.A. and Feneley, R.C.L. (1982) Endorphins – a role in lower urinary tract function? The effect of opioid blockade on the detrusor and urethral sphincter mechanisms. *Br J Urol* **54**, 638–40

Norton, K.R.W., Bhat, A.V. and Stanton, S.L. (1990) Psychiatric aspects of urinary incontinence in women attending an outpatient urodynamic clinic. *BMJ* **301**, 271–2

Oldenburg, B. and Millard, R.J. (1986) Predictors of long-term outcome following a bladder re-training programme. *J Psychosom Res* **30**, 691–4

Pedersen, E. (1977) Studies on the effect and mode of action of flavoxate in human urinary bladder and sphincter. *Urol Int* **32**, 202–6

Philp, T., Shah, P.J.R. and Worth, P.H.L. (1988) Acupuncture in the treatment of bladder instability. *Br J Urol* **61**, 490–3

Rew, D.A. and Rundle, J.S.H. (1989) Assessment of the safety of regular DDAVP therapy in primary nocturnal enuresis. *Br J Urol* **63**, 352–3

Riva, D. and Casolati, E. (1984) Oxybutynin chloride in the treatment of female idiopathic bladder instability. Results from double blind treatment. *Clin Exp Obstet Gynecol* **11**, 37–9

Robertson, A.S., Griffiths, C.J., Ramsden, P.D. and Neal, D.E. (1994) Bladder function in healthy volunteers: ambulatory monitoring and conventional urodynamic studies. *Br J Urol* **73**, 242–9

Rud, T., Andersson, K.E. and Ulmsten, U. (1979) Effects of nifedipine in women with unstable bladders. *Urol Int* **34**, 421–3

Song Baozhu, Wang Xiyou (1985) Short term effect of 135 cases of enuresis treated by wrist ankle needling. *J Tradit Chin Med* **5**, 27–8

Tapp, A.J.S., Cardozo, L.D., Versi, E. and Cooper, D. (1990) The treatment of detrusor instability in post-menopausal women with oxybutynin chloride: a double blind placebo controlled study. *Br J Obstet Gynaecol* **97**, 521–6

Thompson, I.M. and Lauvetz, R. (1976) Oxybutynin in bladder spasm, neurogenic bladder, and enuresis. *Urology* **8**, 452–4

Torrens, M.J. and Griffiths, H.B. (1974) The control of the uninhibited bladder by selective sacral neurectomy. *Br J Urol* **46**, 639–44

Van Gool, J.D. and De Jonge, G.A. (1989) Urge syndrome and urge incontinence. *Arch Dis Child* **64**, 1629–34

Walters, M.D., Taylor, S. and Schoenfeld, L.S. (1990) Psychosexual study of women with detrusor instability. *Obstet Gynecol* **75**, 22–5

Wein, A.J. (1990) Pharmacologic treatment of incontinence. *J Am Geriatr Soc* **30**, 317–25

Whitehead, J.A. (1967) Urinary incontinence in the aged: propantheline bromide as an adjunct to treatment. *Geriatrics* **22**, 154–7

15

Electrical stimulation, a non-surgical means of cure for stress and urge incontinence

Magnus Fall and Sivert Lindström

Introduction

In principle, *urge incontinence* is caused by some type of nervous dysfunction affecting the inhibitory control of the micturition reflex. Functional electrical stimulation (FES) may restore inhibition by artificial activation of normally silent bladder inhibitory reflexes. Defective closure of the urethra may have a variety of causes. Inadequate urethral support is a common factor in *genuine female stress urinary incontinence.* So is inadequate function of the pelvic floor muscle complex, owing to focal, peripheral nerve damage, lack of use or otherwise impaired neuronal control. Voluntary pelvic floor exercise or FES may restore sphincter control and continence when the main cause is a dysfunction of the striated muscles of the pelvic floor. Surgical correction is demanded when urethral hypermobility due to lack of urethral support is the dominating mechanism.

A common therapeutic problem is that stress urinary incontinence is often combined with urgency or urge incontinence, so-called *mixed incontinence*. In such cases, control of the bladder overactivity may be as vital as an improvement of the urethral closure. Electrical stimulation can control both components of incontinence and may therefore be an ideal option.

Physiologic aspects of continence relevant to electrical stimulation

Most striated muscles of the body are composed of three motor unit types, one with slowly contracting muscle fibres and two with fast contraction properties. The intramural urethral sphincter is composed of slow fibres only, whereas the paraurethral striated muscles have varying proportions of all three types. The three motor unit types differ with respect to their maximal force development, fusion frequency and resistance to fatigue. The slow units develop little force but are resistant to fatigue. Their fusion frequency is about 10 Hz, whereas the fastest units can produce 10–20 times more contraction force but fatigue rapidly. Their fusion frequency is around 40–50 Hz. The intermediate fast units are somewhat weaker but considerably more fatigue resistant. These characteristics imply that the intramural striated sphincter can generate a well-sustained but rather limited increase in urethral pressure. Its main function seems to be to accomplish urethral closure during bladder filling at rest, when there is little physical stress. In more provocative situations, when the intra-abdominal pressure suddenly increases, e.g. at lifting, coughing and running (when most women with stress urinary incontinence leak), the fast motor units of the paraurethral pelvic floor muscles are most important. They provide a rapidly induced, strong closing force upon the urethra. There are indications that functional loss of muscle function may be caused by focal damage of the nerve supply to the pelvic floor, resulting in urinary and faecal incontinence (Snooks and Swash 1984). Childbirth seems to be a major precipitating factor for denervation in the female (Allen *et al.* 1990).

It has been shown that the effect of stimulation on the urethra is mediated by activation of somatic nerves to the striated muscles. In clinical experiments, adequate urethral closure was obtained at 20–50 Hz, the lower frequency being a good compromise for patients with mixed stress and urge incontinence. From animal experiments it seems that direct stimulation of efferent fibres is the most important mechanism (Fall *et al.* 1978). A study with single fibre recording in man has emphasised the importance of reflex activation of the motor fibres (Trontelj *et al.* 1974). In this investigation direct responses to stimulation were elicited but reflex responses with a latency of 35 ms or more dominated quantitatively. It has to be noted, though, that the pudendo–pudendal reflex is very frequency sensitive. It may be completely suppressed after a few stimuli with frequencies as low as 2–5 Hz, whereas in clinical studies higher frequencies have always been used, typically 20–100 Hz. Another factor of importance is muscle fatigue. When using FES for incontinence, intermittent trains of impulses have been found to reduce this problem. Intermittent stimulation has been standard in most devices for treatment of incontinence. In clinical practice, the possibility remains that reflex responses are elicited by the first one or two pulses in each train but not the following.

Bladder filling results in activation of mechanoreceptors in the bladder wall. These receptors respond both to passive distension and to active contraction of the detrusor (Lindström *et al.* 1984). The afferent signals are transmitted, mainly via the pelvic nerves, to the spinal cord and ascend bilaterally in the dorso-lateral white matter. The information eventually reaches the cerebral cortex in the medial region of its somatosensory area and gives rise to the sensation of bladder filling and urgency. The afferent signal also influences neurones in Barrington's micturition centre in the upper pons. When appropriately activated, descending neurones in this centre drive preganglionic bladder pelvic neurones in the sacral cord and thereby induce a micturition contraction.

Once initiated the micturition reflex is enhanced by a positive feedback mechanism. The reflex detrusor contraction generates an increased bladder pressure and a further activation of bladder mechanoreceptors. This afference, in turn, reinforces the activation of the pontine micturition centre and the pelvic motor output to the bladder, resulting in increase in bladder pressure and mechanoreceptor afference etc. When urine enters the urethra, the reflex is further enhanced by activation of urethral receptors (Barrington 1914). Normally, this positive feedback mechanism ascertains a complete emptying of the bladder during micturition. A drawback with this kind of arrangement is that the reflex system may easily become unstable. Any stimulus that activates the mechanoreceptor afferents may trigger a micturition reflex. To prevent this during bladder filling, the micturition reflex pathway is controlled by several inhibitory mechanisms at spinal and supraspinal levels.

Appropriate functional electrical stimulation activates inhibitory pathways to the micturition reflex, without a general effect on receptor systems and consequently without general side-effects. Penile, clitoral and vaginal electrical stimulation activates a reflex with its afferent limb in the pudendal nerve and with three concomitant central actions: activation of hypogastric inhibitory fibres to the bladder, central inhibition of the pelvic outflow to the bladder and central inhibition of the ascending afferent pathway from the bladder. This reflex is silent at rest and seems to be designed to prevent bladder contractions during coitus. Anal stimulation inhibits the bladder in a similar fashion by a reflex with its afferent limb in pelvic nerve branches to the anal region, a reflex designed to inhibit the bladder during defecation. Thus, perineal methods for electrical stimulation utilise natural reflexes that are silent during normal, everyday life but capable of sustained bladder inhibition when evoked by continuous or intermittent electrical stimulation.

Clinical practice of electrical stimulation

The first clinical trials of electrical stimulation were started in the beginning of the 1960s by Caldwell and co-workers (Caldwell 1963). They used a device for implantation with electrodes situated in the pelvic floor muscles, activated from a subcutaneous receiver and antenna. Implantation involves the risks of major surgery and problems with the durability of the implanted device. Other investigators tried external devices and obtained equally good results. In all early trials low-intensity, long-term home stimulation procedures were utilised. These systems require a very long period of treatment to give clinical effects, several hours of stimulation per day or night during several months, a procedure putting demands on the motivation and persistence of the patient to continue treatment. In this context it also has to be remembered that many of the early devices used electrodes with a suboptimal mechanical fitness. Unfortunately, no ideal electrode carrier is yet commercially available. Subsequently, a different procedure was introduced, referred to as acute maximal functional stimulation (AMFES) or simply maximal stimulation (Godec and Cass 1978). In this routine the patient is stimulated for 20–30 minutes at maximum tolerable intensity, preferably using combinations of vaginal-anal-penile/ cutaneous electrodes. The treatment has to be repeated, usually 4–10 times or more during a 2–3 week period.

Long-term and maximal stimulation procedures probably utilise the same neurophysiological mechanisms. In long-term treatment the more comfortable intensity has to be compensated for by a considerably longer treatment period, whereas in maximal stimulation the gain in treatment time has to be paid for by a more unpleasant stimulation. A practical compromise between the two modalities is so-called home-maximal stimulation administered by a personal device for home treatment, giving higher intensity than the conventional long-term stimulator and thereby permitting shorter sequences of stimulation (Plevnik et al. 1986). The results in several series of patients presented, treated with different modalities of electrical stimulation, are surprisingly consistent. About 80% of patients are cured or improved (Fall et al. 1994).

Despite the large body of clinical experience, including a large number of centres producing rather impressive clinical results in different categories of incontinent patients, there has been a slow acceptance of electrical stimulation, a major argument being the lack of controlled studies. In this context it should be emphasised that several facts speak in favour of a 'real' effect of stimulation:

1 The physiologic observations mentioned above are a very strong argument to support the clinical efficacy of electrical stimulation in overactive bladder and sphincter weakness.
2 The proportion of improved and cured patients clearly exceeds an expected placebo effect. The rate of improvement cannot be ascribed entirely to such a mechanism because of the consistancy and level of success in the different materials so far presented.
3 A re-education effect lasting for up to five years has been reported. This kind of effect has not been documented in drug studies (including placebo) on comparable materials of patients. Still, controlled studies would be desirable to determine the level of the placebo effect. The lack of a good placebo equivalent to active treatment is a major obstacle when trying to design such a trial.

Two factors are essential for the successful practice of electrical stimulation treatment:

1 Therapy has to be restricted to categories of patients in whom stimulation has a documented effect: detrusor instability rather than urgency of undefined or sensory character, stress incontinence due to sphincter weakness rather than caused by a defunctionalised urethra or excessive urethral hypermobility, respectively.
2 If treatment is administered by a personal device to be used at home, the counselling of the patient is the key to a good result. Especially during the initial period there is need for support to motivate the patient but in our experience little back-up is necessary during continuing treatment; our drop-out rate has been very small. The initial device training is crucial for the outcome of therapy. Preferably, the person who has supervised the training should answer the questions. The ideal person for this is a specially trained nurse or incontinence adviser.

Conclusion

Electrical stimulation is simple, cheap, non-destructive, has few side-effects and can be used in different types of incontinence, with a potential curative effect. Although there is a need for further technical development and improved knowledge about the mechanisms of re-education, the physiological effects on the striated muscles and the magnitude of the placebo effect, electrical stimulation has great potential but is clearly underevaluated at present.

Acknowledgement

The authors were supported by the Swedish Medical Research Council, project numbers 9902 and 4767.

References

Allen, R.E., Hosker, G.L., Smith, A.R.B. *et al.* (1990) Pelvic floor damage and childbirth: a neurophysiological study. *Br J Obstet Gynaecol* **97**, 770–9

Barrington, F.J.F. (1914) The nervous control of micturition. *Q J Exp Physiol* **8**. 33–71

Caldwell, K.P.S. (1963) The electrical control of sphincter incompetence. *Lancet* **2**, 174–5

Fall, M. and Madersbacher, H. (1994) 'Peripheral electrical stimulation' in Mundy, Stephenson and Wein (Eds). *Urodynamics: Principles, Practice and Application* (2nd ed.) Edinburgh: Churchill-Livingstone

Fall, M., Erlandson, B.-E., Carlsson, C.-A. *et al.* (1978) The effect of intravaginal electrical stimulation on the feline urethra and urinary bladder: neuronal mechanisms. *Scand J Urol Nephrol* **44** (suppl), 19–30

Godec, C. and Cass, A.S. (1978) Acute electrical stimulation for urinary incontinence. *Urology* **12**, 340–2

Lindström, S., Fall, M., Carlsson, C.-A. *et al.* (1984) Rhythmic activity in pelvic efferents to the bladder: an experimental study in the cat with reference to the clinical condition 'unstable bladder'. *Urol Int* **39**, 272–9

Plevnik, S., Janez, J., Vrtacnik, P. *et al.* (1986) Short-term electrical stimulation: home treatment for urinary incontinence. *World J Urol* **4**, 24–6

Snooks, S.H. and Swash, M. (1984) Abnormalities of the innervation of the urethral striated sphincter musculature in incontinence. *Br J Urol* **56**, 401–6

Trontelj, J.V., Janko, M., Godec, C. *et al.* (1974) Electrical stimulation for urinary incontinence. *Urol Int* **29**, 213–20

16

Voiding difficulties and retention

Julian Shah

Introduction

Normal voiding takes place by initiation of bladder contraction with simultaneous relaxation of the bladder neck and urethra. The act of micturition is determined by a number of separate factors: control from higher centres, the sacral reflex arc, the innervation of the bladder muscle and sphincter mechanisms, the outflow resistance and the speed of contraction of the detrusor muscle fibres. If there are abnormalities present in any part of this complex mechanism, a voiding disorder may develop.

Voiding disorders in the female are common but too often go unrecognised until the patient presents with symptoms which are troublesome, such as recurrent urinary tract infection or incontinence. Difficulty with micturition may not be as noticeable to the female as she may not be aware of the rate of a change in the rate of urine flow. Competitive voiding which is a natural accompaniment of male development, is not found in the female! Normal voiding is accomplished without straining. However, some normal females occasionally void by straining. Increases in flow rate may be achieved by a rise in intra-abdominal pressure in the female because of the lower outflow resistance within the short female urethra. Female voiding occurs at a higher flow rate and at a lower voiding pressure than the male. It is not unusual to observe, during videocystometry, rapid and efficient voiding taking place with no rise in intravesical pressure. This phenomenon is not due to the fact that the urine 'just falls out', as it is sometimes said, but because a very low resistance requires a very low pressure to overcome it. If these bladders are observed during voiding on videocystometry they can be seen to be contracting very efficiently. The speed of contraction of these low-pressure bladders is normal, the tension in the bladder muscle fibres is low and thus the voiding pressure is low. These low-pressure bladders tend to have little reserve and are more prone to develop voiding difficulty if the outflow resistance is increased. The majority of patients with low pressure but efficient voiding who have surgery for stress incontinence may have initial difficulty with voiding demonstrated by incomplete bladder emptying. In some, this may be asymptomatic. Almost all of these bladders return to satisfactory emptying within a month after surgery.

Definitions

It is worth while having a simple definition for each of the commonly encountered voiding disorders which will ensure that all clinicians refer to the same conditions with the same terminology (see Table 16.1).

Table 16.1   Classification of voiding difficulties and retention

Condition	Symptom	Urodynamic data
Asymptomatic voiding difficulty	Frequency Urgency due to urinary infection, or No symptoms	Obstructed flow Elevated, normal or reduced voiding pressure ± Residual urine or large capacity with low pressure voiding
Symptomatic voiding difficulty	Poor stream Incomplete emptying Straining Frequency	Flow <15 ml/sec Elevated voiding pressure >50 cm H_2O ± Residual urine
Acute retention	Painful or painless sudden onset	Residual urine
Chronic retention	Reduced sensation Hesitancy Straining to void Frequency, nocturia Urgency, incontinence Urinary tract infection	Flow <15 ml/sec Residual urine High pressure or low pressure voiding
Acute-on-chronic retention	Painful or painless sudden onset History of chronic retention Incontinence	Residual urine

Acute retention is the sudden onset of the inability to void. This may be either painful (where neurology is normal) or painless (where abnormal neurology is present). Acute retention usually occurs over a period of 4–6 hours but may be present for longer periods if the patient does not present earlier. A volume equal to or greater than normal capacity is removed by catheterisation (usually 500 ml or more) (see Table 16.2).

Chronic retention is difficult to define as different clinicians may have different opinions as to its nature. It is worth while remembering that normal bladders do not retain residual urine (Shah *et al.* 1981) It is quite logical to consider that retained residual volume of 50 ml must be associated with a voiding dysfunction. Though this may be true, a generally acceptable definition of chronic retention is not available. One possible definition is that chronic retention is present when the bladder constantly retains a volume equal to its normal capacity (e.g. approximately 500 ml) and the bladder is painlessly enlarged and usually palpable. Bladders that do not normally empty completely and leave any residual urine on a regular basis are abnormal and the definition of chronic retention is one of degree. Chronic retention may be a cause of urinary incontinence because of overflow and may occur without any known aetiology (Deane and Worth 1985; Fox *et al.* 1976).

Many patients may have a voiding disorder of which they are unaware. Even the presence of severe abnormalities of bladder emptying may be accepted as normal for an individual if there is no means of comparison. This is more likely in the

Table 16.2   Causes of acute retention in the female

Post-operative	– Rectal surgery
	– Hysterectomy
	– Surgery for stress incontinence
	– After any surgical procedure
Neurological	– Multiple sclerosis
	– Myelitis
	– Diabetes mellitus
Gynaecological	– Uterine prolapse
	– Cystocele
Urethral calculus	
Urethral stricture	
Acute cystitis	
Rectal constipation	
Psychogenic	
Idiopathic	

female, for reasons already stated. The likely sequence of events in a patient with urethral obstruction will be that of raised intravesical pressure with normal flow to be followed by raised intravesical pressure and reduced pressure and eventually that of bladder 'decompensation' with low pressure/low flow voiding and residual urine. As many as 14% of females that presented to a urodynamic clinic with bladder symptoms were shown to have voiding disorders (Stanton *et al.* 1985).

Aetiology and pathophysiology

There are many causes of voiding disorders in the female. Abnormalities of voiding function may be due to interruption of the normal voiding reflex which occurs in neurological disease, failure of detrusor contraction or to an abnormality of urethral function. Habit and psychological factors may also be involved. The many causes of voiding dysfunction are listed in Table 16.3.

Neurological disorders

Lesions in the nervous system tend to produce specific types of voiding abnormality.

Lesions in the brain which affect voiding function may occur in the frontal lobes, internal capsule, reticular formation of the pons and cerebellum. These abnormalities will tend to vary according to the severity of the lesion, the age of the patient and whether dementia forms part of the neurological process. Voiding disorders that are associated with confusional states in the elderly often right themselves once the confusional state is corrected. Urinary retention may result from acute lesions such as cerebrovascular accidents whereas more chronic lesions such as multiple sclerosis

Table 16.3   Causes of voiding difficulties and retention

1   *Neurological disease*
     As a result of spinal injury – spinal shock phase
     Upper motor neurone lesion – spinal injury, multiple sclerosis
     Lower motor neurone lesion – spinal injury, multiple sclerosis
     Autonomic lesion – e.g. after pelvic surgery
     Local pain reflex after surgery

2   *Pharmacological*
     Tricyclic antidepressants
     Anticholinergic agents
        – adrenergic agents
     Ganglion blocking agents
     Epidural anaesthesia

3   *Acute inflammation*
     Acute urethritis
     Acute cystitis
     Acute vulvovaginitis
     Acute ano–genital infection (including herpes)

4   *Obstruction*
     Distal urethral stenosis
     Acute urethral oedema of surgery
     Chronic urethral stenosis
     Foreign body or calculus in the urethra
     Impacted pelvic mass – retroverted gravid uterus
                          – haematocolpos
                          – uterine fibroid
                          – ovarian cyst
                          – faecal impaction
     Urethral distortion with cystocele
     Ectopic ureterocele
     Uterine prolapse
     Leiomyoma of the bladder

5   *Endocrine*
     Hypothyroidism
     Diabetic neuropathy

6   *Overdistension*

7   *Psychogenic*
     Anxiety or depressive illness
     Hysteria

8   *Iatrogenic*
     After transtrigonal phenol injections
     After surgery for stress incontinence
     After anal surgery
     After hysterectomy

9   *Idiopathic*

and Parkinson's disease may be associated with detrusor hyper-reflexia and its consequences of urinary frequency, urgency and incontinence.

Lesions in the spinal cord may be caused by trauma, tumours, prolapse of an intervertebral disc or spina bifida. If the lesion is above the sacral parasympathetic reflex arc, after a period of spinal shock (which occurs after acute spinal cord insult), the bladder becomes autonomous and its urodynamic dysfunction is represented by hyper-reflexic detrusor behaviour combined with detrusor sphincter dyssynergia. This combination almost invariably leads to urinary incontinence in the female, often combined with the retention of varying degrees of residual urine due to the unco-ordinated relationship between detrusor and sphincter function.

Lesions which occur below the reflex arc at or below the level of the outlet of the sacral roots tend to produce bladder acontractility. This type of bladder dysfunction produces a bladder that does not contract (acontractile), with an associated non-relaxing sphincter mechanism. These patients tend to void by straining, often leaving a residual urine, though incontinence may be a feature due to chronic retention with overflow.

Pelvic plexus injuries occur as a result of damage to the pelvic plexus nerves during surgical procedures in the pelvis, such as abdomino–perineal excision of the rectum or radical hysterectomy. The neurological lesion may be incomplete and produces a disorder of bladder function which is unpredictable. A bladder with reduced compliance, urinary incontinence and incomplete emptying may result.

A pelvic nerve injury may also rarely follow the transtrigonal injection of the pelvic plexus nerves with phenol for the treatment of detrusor instability (Cox and Worth 1984).

Pharmacological causes

The use of anticholinergic agents, of which there are now many in general, may cause voiding dysfunction. The most commonly prescribed agents are atropine (used in premedication), probanthine, oxybutynin, imipramine and other tricyclic antidepressants. All these agents have potent anticholinergic effects which reduce the power of bladder contraction. If used for the treatment of detrusor instability or detrusor hyper-reflexia they usually produce beneficial reduction in voiding frequency and incontinence. However, if used in the presence of undiagnosed detrusor hypofunction these agents may be responsible for the weakening of detrusor power and varying degrees of retention. In spinal injury units anticholinergic agents are used to produce retention so that continence may result. Bladder drainage is then by intermittent catheterisation.

Ganglion blocking agents produce similar effects to the anticholinergic drugs, whilst alpha-stimulants increase outflow resistance and consequent voiding dysfunction.

Epidural anaesthesia may produce temporary retention by interruption of the reflex arc.

Acute inflammation

Acute inflammation of the urethra, vulva, vagina or bladder may be associated with urinary retention or abnormalities of bladder emptying with frequency of micturition, obstructed flow and incomplete bladder emptying. If the acute inflammatory process produces urethral oedema this will increase the outflow resistance.

Genital herpes affecting the ano-genital region (Oates and Greenhouse 1978) and affecting the cervix or vulva (Hemrika *et al.* 1986; Ryttov *et al.* 1985) have been shown to cause acute urinary retention. The urinary effects are thought to be due to central nervous involvement with the likeliest lesion being a lumbosacral meningomyelitis. However, any painful vulvo–vaginal lesion may contribute to voiding dysfunction.

Obstruction

Bladder outflow obstruction in the normal female is usually a consequence of failure of relaxation of the urethral sphincter mechanism. In the female with neuropathy, this tends to be due to detrusor sphincter dyssynergia.

The diagnosis of urethral stenosis in the female is uncommon; a urologist may expect to see very few true urethral stenoses each year. It is usually the result of urethral scarring following chronic urethral inflammation, in association with surgery around the urethra, or as a consequence of instrumentation. Typically the condition occurs in the postmenopausal woman and there is no obvious aetiological cause. Occasionally a urethral caruncle may be associated with urethral stenosis or its surgical treatment may cause stenosis. The diagnosis of urethral stenosis is made at the time of urethral catheterisation, at cystometry or cystography, or at endoscopy to diagnose voiding difficulty. Urethral stenosis is treated by urethral dilatation, either by means of graduated urethral dilators or the Otis urethrotome.

Other causes of urethral obstruction include urethral oedema secondary to premenstrual fluid retention and foreign bodies within the urethra, including urethral calculi.

Impaction of a retroverted gravid uterus, uterine fibroids and ovarian cysts may all cause retention of urine. A haematocolpos may also cause retention if impacted in the pelvis. An ectopic ureterocele may be a rare cause of voiding dysfunction in children.

A large cystocele with descent of the bladder neck may cause urethral distortion or 'kinking' which may produce a functional obstruction. Repair of the cystocele may then be all that is necessary to restore the normal continuity of the urethra and normal voiding. This underlines the importance of vaginal examination in all females with voiding difficulties.

Surgery for stress incontinence is associated with abnormalities of bladder emptying. Although repositioning of the bladder neck into an intra-abdominal environment is the primary aim of the modern surgical treatment of stress incontinence in the female, there is sufficient evidence to suggest that voiding difficulty is a consequence of both vaginal and abdominal procedures. The Burch colposuspension produces a high lift to the bladder neck with consequent stretching of the urethra especially if the vaginal sutures are tied closely to the pectineal ligament. It should be expected that these patients may experience voiding problems after surgery (Walter *et al.* 1982; Stanton and Cardozo 1983; Lose *et al.* 1987). Those patients with pre-operative low pressure voiding are particularly likely to run into difficulty with bladder emptying in the early post-operative phase. All but a small percentage of

Table 16.4 Urodynamic diagnoses in females with a hypersensitive urethra and the symptoms of frequency, nocturia and urgency of micturition

Urodynamic diagnosis	Hypersensitive urethral state	Normal urethras
n =	50	50
Detrusor instability	14 (28%)	36 (72%)
Normal detrusor function	36 (72%)	14 (28%)
Obstructed	15 (30%)	6 (12%)
Stress incontinence	15 (30%)	12 (24%)

these patients will recover normal bladder emptying but usually with reduced flow rates.

After endoscopic bladder neck suspension (Stamey 1972), voiding difficulties do occur (Coptcoat and Shah 1988). Although some authorities claim that normal voiding continues after this form of surgery, it is not unreasonable to suggest that part of the successful result of this type of surgery is the consequence of increasing the resistance within the urethra as well as the repositioning effect.

As well as those iatrogenic causes mentioned above which may be partly or entirely responsible for voiding dysfunction, anal surgery (Lyngdorf *et al.* 1986) and other factors listed in Table 16.2 may be involved and should be carefully considered in the aetiology if the primary cause is not immediately obvious.

The hypersensitive female urethra

There is a group of female patients with the symptoms of frequency, nocturia and urgency who, when undergoing urodynamic investigations, are found at the time of catheterisation to have exquisitely sensitive urethras (Shah *et al.* 1981). The results of urodynamic study in these patients reveals a lower incidence of detrusor instability and a high incidence of obstructed voiding when compared with a similar group of females with the same symptoms but normal urethras (Table 16.4). The hypersensitive urethra probably represents an inflammatory condition of unknown aetiology which gives rise to the symptoms mentioned. Urethral dilatation using the Otis urethrotome appears to provide some of these patients with relief. A cause for the inflammatory process should be sought.

Overdistension

Bladder overdistension should never be overlooked as a potent cause of voiding disturbance. After surgical procedures such as hysterectomy, or during delivery, any retention should be relieved immediately. I have seen patients who, after a single episode of urinary retention of several hours, have not recovered normal voiding function and are left with hypo or acontractile bladders. This should sound a note of caution. If a female patient cannot void it is far better to pass a small-bore catheter to relieve the retention as soon as possible. Ignoring the patient's symptoms is not acceptable as the patient is usually correct. If the retention is relieved quickly the patient is very grateful and a long-term voiding problem will be avoided. The patient may void in a hot bath or shower which does assist pelvic floor and general relaxation but if the bladder is significantly overdistended this may not be successful. Drugs to stimulate bladder contraction are often unsuccessful and carry their own risks and side-effects and have been shown to carry no significant benefit.

Psychogenic retention

This diagnosis should only be made when, after a careful process of exclusion, no abnormalities have been discovered. The occasional late neurological abnormality may turn up in an initially apparently normal patient. A careful history and examination is necessary along with a neurological examination performed by a neurologist. The majority of patients suffering from psychogenic retention of urine are females aged between 15 and 45 years. There is usually a relationship between the onset of the retention and a stressful event such as childbirth, marital discord, surgical treatment or rape (Krane and Siroky 1900). Hysteria, depression, and schizophrenia may all be causes of this problem. However, once a psychiatric diagnosis is made the treatment remains the same as in normal patients. Return to normal voiding function may be expected in the majority (Barrett 1978), though the use of clean intermittent catheterisation for each of these patients is satisfactory management.

Presentation

Symptoms

Many females are infrequent voiders. That is to say that they may void only once or twice a day. Some patients with disorders of voiding function may not be aware that they have a problem until they develop urinary tract infection or retention. Bladder inflammation is common in the female, occurring in childhood in association with abnormalities of the urinary tract, in young adult life in association with sexual intercourse, in middle age with the menopause and in the elderly in association with urinary tract pathology such as tumours, calculi and chronic inflammation. The young adult female should be questioned about voiding difficulty if infection occurs. A free flow rate will generally exclude an obstructive problem.

Lower urinary tract infection in an older female should be investigated more completely as abnormalities of bladder function are more likely.

Females will admit to the symptom of poor stream. Straining to void is associated with reduced contractility of the detrusor. A feeling of incomplete emptying may be associated with retained residual urine. Urinary frequency may occur with chronic retention leading to urinary incontinence as an outflow phenomenon although this is uncommon in the female.

A general history with particular reference to past medical and surgical treatment is very important as many voiding problems stem from or are temporarily related to previous pelvic and abdominal surgery and childbirth. A drug history should also be obtained.

Signs

Examination of the urinary tract is often felt to be unrewarding. It is all the more important therefore that a careful general, abdominal and pelvic examination should be undertaken. The kidneys should be carefully palpated and are usually felt in all but the very obese. Abdominal masses should be noted. It is not always easy to palpate the full bladder during abdominal examination. Bimanual examination will often confirm one's suspicions of bladder fullness as the bladder may be more easily palpable. Gentle percussion in the suprapubic region will reveal the characteristic dullness which is present when the bladder is full or when other pelvic masses are present.

The importance of clinical examination cannot be overemphasised and this particularly applies to the wheelchair-bound patient who is particularly difficult to examine because of immobility and deformity. When examining this group of patients one often discovers the most severe abnormalities.

The urethra should be examined for its appearance, position and tenderness. Urethral tenderness can be assessed by its compression against the back of the pubic symphysis. The normal female urethra is not tender. The vulva and vagina should be observed for signs of hormonal withdrawal and inflammation, for prolapse and scarring in association with childbirth and previous surgery. A careful bimanual examination should also be made.

A general neurological examination should be performed, though if a neurological abnormality is suspected a neurologist's opinion should be sought. The patient's general demeanour should also be observed.

Investigation

Investigations should be used sensibly. The patient should be investigated according to the suspected abnormality. It is unacceptable to use inappropriate investigations because of lack of knowledge and experience. As these patients' symptoms are related to the lower urinary tract, it is quite unnecessary to perform urography. The simplest tests available are a flow rate, abdominal radiograph (to look for calcification and soft tissue masses) and pelvic and, if appropriate, renal ultrasonography. The demonstration of a reduced flow and a residual urine on bladder ultrasound will confirm a diagnosis of voiding difficulty and the next step will be to perform urodynamic studies.

The frequency/volume voided chart or urinary diary

If the patient is referred with a voiding problem, useful information will be obtained by asking the patient to keep a urinary diary for one week prior to attending for consultation. A standard diary sheet should be sent to the patient with the outpatient appointment and the patient given instructions on how to fill it in. Even the most elderly patient will not find this task difficult. A record of fluid intake, volumes voided and the timing of voids, episodes of incontinence and any other relevant features may then be discussed with the patient. These charts are also later valuable for the assessment of the response to therapy (Giesy 1986).

Infrequent voiding

Why we void the number of times we do is determined by a number of factors. It is important to be aware of these factors so that pathological changes which do occur may be recognised. Normal voiding frequency, generally accepted as less than seven times daily, is determined by fluid intake, habit, anxiety and stress, and the presence of abnormalities of bladder function which may be motor or sensory. Infrequent voiding, i.e. the passing of urine less than two or three times a day with a normal fluid intake is abnormal. Patients who void infrequently should be investigated at least with a frequency/intake output/volume voided chart and, based upon the information obtained, advised about their normal requirements of intake and the frequency of voiding. Infrequent voiders should be recommended to void every 3–4 hours during the day. Infrequent voiding with normal bladder volumes should not lead to long-term bladder harm.

The flow rate

The free urine flow rate is the simplest and possibly most useful urodynamic investigation, particularly because it is non-invasive. Every department that is involved with the management of urinary disorders should be equipped with a flow machine which may be purchased at a cost of £1000–2000. The use of such equipment will more than pay for itself because of its value in saving patients from unnecessary investigations and treatment. The flow machine should be kept in a private area, preferably a toilet, so that the patient may void in privacy. This reduces the erroneous flows that may be seen when the patient is inhibited or embarrassed.

A series of flow rates obtained on a single day with bladder volumes greater than 200 ml demonstrates the benefit of the flow rate clinic. A single flow rate is not sufficient for providing a true indication of flow and three consecutive flow rates should be obtained. The patient should be asked to void when full but not to hold on too long. Flow rates should be obtained with voided volumes of 200 ml or more, though flow rate values will fall within the normal range (in normal females) when small volumes are passed (Figure 16.1). If the volume voided is persistently small the pattern of the flow curve should be examined carefully. If the volume voided is less than 200 ml an artefactually low flow rate may be recorded and give rise to misinterpretation. The superimposition of a number of flow curves in the same female demonstrate that except when the volumes are very small or very large the flow curves are very similar (Figure 16.2).

A normal flow rate is seen in Figure 16.3. Examples of abnormal flow patterns are shown in Figures 16.4 and 16.5. The normal flow rate depends upon: (a) volume voided, and (b) age. As ageing progresses the flow rate values tend to fall. Abrams and Torrens (1979) quote the following lower limits for flow rate at different ages:

under 50 years: >25 ml/sec
over 50 years: >18 ml/sec

Obstructed voiding may occur even in the presence of normal flowmetry. This is because the bladder has been able to compensate through an increase in the force of contraction associated with a rise in voiding pressure. In these patients it is

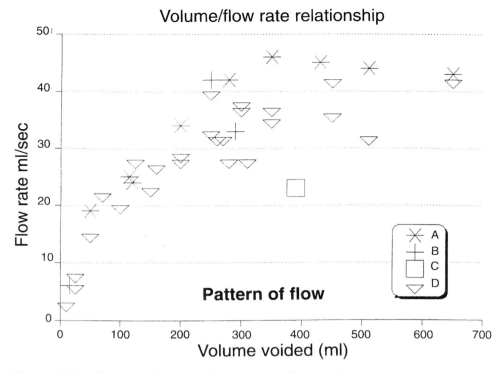

Figure 16.1 Flow rates in normal females according to volumes voided

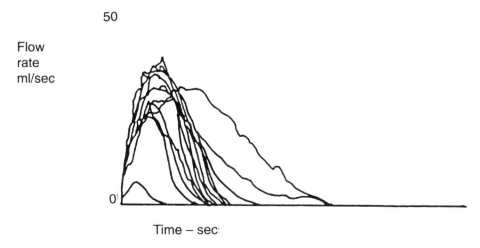

Figure 16.2 Flow rates at different volumes in a normal female to demonstrate the uniformity of the flow curves except where bladder volumes are either very small or very large

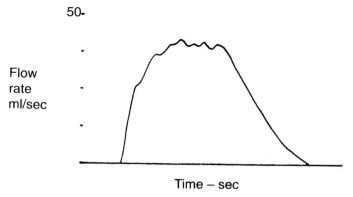

Figure 16.3   Normal flow rate in a female

important to listen carefully to the symptom complex and if obstructed voiding is present, in spite of normal flowmetry, urodynamic evaluation is indicated.

Urethral pressure profilometry

Profilometry does not contribute to the diagnosis and management of voiding disorders. Perhaps in the absence of electromyography this technique may have some usefulness in the investigation of neuropathy or suspected 'voluntary' external striated sphincter dyssynergia, though simultaneous cystometry and intra-urethral pressure recording should be used in these cases both during filling and voiding.

Cystometry

Urodynamic investigation will provide the most clinically useful information in this group of patients and should always be used where there is doubt about the diagnosis and always where neuropathy may be the cause of the voiding problem. Filling and voiding cystometry may be all that is necessary for the majority of patients; however, combined synchronous videocystometry is preferable where available, especially where neuropathic disorders are known or suspected. Videocystometry enables radiological examination of the voiding process and will provide information about the bladder appearance – the presence or absence of trabeculation, diverticula and reflux, and the behaviour of the bladder neck and urethral mechanisms. External striated sphincter function should be carefully examined during videocystometry. Abnormalities of sphincter function are seen in some normal patients who have inhibited voiding and in neuropathic disorders where detrusor sphincter dyssynergia gives rise to obstructed voiding. Table 16.5 describes the features which may be encountered in the urodynamic investigation of voiding dysfunction.

Urodynamic findings according to the disorder

Acute retention – If the primary cause is known and its treatment successful, urodynamic investigation will not be necessary.

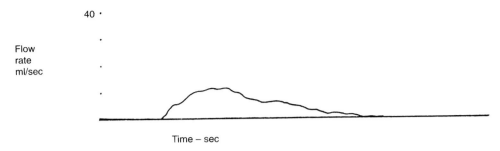

Figure 16.4   Low flow due to outflow obstruction

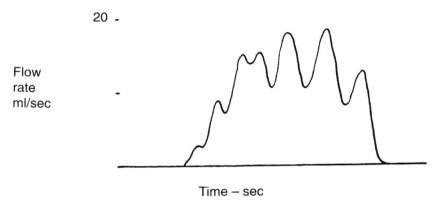

Figure 16.5   Intermittent flow associated with hypocontractile detrusor function and straining to void

Chronic retention – may be due to a complete failure of detrusor function. If this is the case, urodynamics will demonstrate a large capacity, low pressure bladder during filling, with little or no detrusor contraction during voiding (acontractile or hypocontractile voiding detrusor function).

If chronic retention is related to obstruction, urodynamic study may demonstrate a high voiding detrusor pressure, low flow rate and with or without residual urine. If, however, it is related to neuropathy, the retention of residual urine is either due to a lower motor neurone lesion with detrusor acontractility or to obstructed detrusorhyper-reflexia (detrusor sphincter dyssynergia). Videocystometry is particularly important in this group of patients. Practically the only female patients who develop upper urinary tract dilatation in association with abnormalities of bladder function are those with neuropathic bladder disorders, where high pressure contractions, detrusor sphincter dyssynergia and residual urine under pressure due to poor bladder compliance occur.

Disorders of voiding function – For *obstructed voiding*, flow rate and post-micturition bladder ultrasound should be carried out initially, followed by videocystometry to confirm the site of obstruction.

Table 16.5   Urodynamic features of voiding disorders

Residual urine >50 ml

First sensation may be greatly reduced or delayed; may be associated with early first sensation and urgency in upper motor neurone lesions

Capacity reduced with hyper-reflexic bladder dysfunction; increased with acontractile bladders

End-filling detrusor pressure and compliance usually normal except in association with upper motor neurone hyper-reflexic bladders or chronic bladder fibrosis

Isometric pressure (Piso) – the additional detrusor pressure rise seen at the point of maximum detrusor pressure during voiding when voiding is suddenly stopped. The Piso tends to relate to detrusor reserve. In patients with low pressure voiding the Piso may be non-existant. Females with low isometric pressures and low voiding pressures tend to be those who take longer to recover normal bladder emptying after surgery for stress incontinence

Maximum voiding pressure
Voiding pressure is raised above the female upper limit of accepted normality (50 cm H$_2$O) where obstruction is present.
Voiding pressure may be low or non-existant where detrusor failure is present

Detrusor failure or denervation with hypocontractility should be investigated by cystometry with the provision of a private voiding facility where pressure flow studies may be performed with the least patient inhibition.

Electromyography (EMG)

The external striated sphincter EMG has a limited place in the investigation of voiding dysfunction. The EMG requires special equipment and considerable experience in its use and interpretation. That is not to say that the EMG should not be employed in the special circumstances in which it is useful, i.e. pelvic floor denervation or suspect but unproven neuropathy.

The EMG may be performed either by needle electrodes placed into the external striated sphincter or by means of an anal plug electrode. Mass sphincter activity will be seen with the latter. Single fibre EMG during which electromyographic activity is recorded on an oscilloscope will demonstrate abnormalities of motor unit activity. Multiphasic motor unit potentials are associated with denervation. Reflex latency times may also be assessed using the EMG and are recommended in patients with unexplained acute retention of urine in whom a neurological abnormality may be present (Fidas *et al.* 1987).

The EMG is associated with discomfort for the patient and in most circumstances videocystometry will provide all the information that is necessary to make a diagnosis which will enable appropriate management. For example a patient with an acontractile bladder of whatever cause will be treated by intermittent catheterisation.

Radiology

Radiological investigations should include a plain abdominal radiograph and where necessary a bladder and upper urinary tract ultrasound scan. Ultrasonography of the pelvic organs may also be helpful in displaying uterine enlargement and ovarian abnormalities. Videocystometry will be used as suggested above. An intravenous urogram is not a dynamic investigation and should not be necessary except where the anatomy of the urinary tract is required. This is rarely necessary in voiding disorders except perhaps again in the hyper-reflexic neuropathic bladder with suspected upper tract dilatation.

Endoscopy

Endoscopy should not be used as a means of diagnosing abnormalities of detrusor function. Obstruction, except for the presence of urethral stenosis, cannot be diagnosed at endoscopy. Endoscopy is necessary for the diagnosis of suspected intravesical abnormalities such as tumours, foreign bodies and stones. It is also used as part of a treatment regime, i.e. in association with urethral dilatation, Otis urethrotomy or repositioning procedures.

Trabeculation which is seen at cystoscopy is common in the female bladder. The very thin female bladder wall may look trabeculated when overdistended. Trabeculation and diverticula are more likely to be associated with detrusor instability than with obstruction (Shah *et al.* 1981).

Trabeculation

Bladder smooth muscle bundles are arranged in a criss-cross or decussating fashion and when affected by hypertrophy are known as trabeculation. Trabeculation may be seen at cystoscopy in the female bladder and in its milder forms may be a part of the range of normal bladder appearances, particularly when the bladder is overdistended.

Trabeculation, however, is generally a sign of developing smooth muscle hypertrophy and its degree varies from very mild to very gross and represents exercise hypertrophy of the smooth muscle bundles. In the late phase of trabeculation the muscle fibres become replaced by connective tissue. Trabeculation may be seen at cystoscopy or on radiological investigations of the bladder, such as urography or cystography. Trabeculation may be caused by outflow obstruction following urethral stenosis or external sphincter dyssynergia, by neuropathic bladder disorders following spinal injury or spina bifida or as a result of detrusor instability. If trabeculation is seen during investigation, detrusor instability and hyper-reflexia are more common causes than obstruction, and this applies both to male and female patients (Shah *et al.* 1981). Gross trabeculation is less common in the female with neuropathy than in the male because the outflow resistance is lower and thus the recurrent effects of isometric detrusor contractions are less marked.

Treatment

Prophylactic measures

Many voiding difficulties may be avoided by the early recognition of potential problems. Therefore if urinary retention is suspected or imminent after surgical procedures, the early use of bladder catheterisation before bladder overdistension has occurred will prevent many long-term bladder problems. If a patient complains of voiding difficulty after surgery, or cannot void, the institution of a programme of intermittent catheterisation until the time of recovery of bladder function is recommended. If the patient will not accept this regime and voiding problems are likely to be prolonged, a suprapubic catheter is recommended.

Difficulty with resuming normal micturition after surgical treatment may occur in over 60% of patients undergoing surgery for stress incontinence (slings, colposuspension and endoscopic bladder neck suspension), and in 45% of patients undergoing radical pelvic surgery (for gynaecological malignancy or after rectal surgery) (Fraser 1966; Smith *et al.* 1969) and after epidural anaesthesia for childbirth or gynaecological procedures. In-dwelling catheters should therefore be used prophylactically after any surgical procedure which may, through a direct or indirect effect, be associated with voiding problems. If the catheter is to be placed for only a short period of time, a urethral catheter of small calibre (e.g. 14 Fr) should be used. However, if a catheter is required for longer periods or if trials of voiding and assessment of bladder emptying, by measurement of residual urine, is necessary a self-retaining suprapubic catheter is preferable.

A clear explanation of the possibility of voiding difficulty should be given to all patients who are to undergo any surgery which carries this risk. Those patients who express dissatisfaction with surgical outcome are those who have not received an adequate pre-operative explanation of the potential problems. It is also very helpful where indicated, to teach the female patient the art of self-catheterisation pre-operatively. If it is not later needed, the patient is very pleased; if it is found necessary, the patient is not aggrieved.

The process of intermittent catheterisation should be a part of the training of both medical and nursing staff involved in the management of these patients.

Intermittent self-catheterisation

Intermittent self-catheterisation was first described by Guttman and Frankel in 1966 for the management of incomplete bladder emptying in the spinal injured patient. Intermittent catheterisation has revolutionised the management of disorders of voiding and enables many women to lead normal lives with efficient bladder emptying, freed from the constraints of struggles with voiding which may involve considerable discomfort, distress and time. It is not unusual to find that a patient with voiding difficulty due to acontractile bladder function may spend several hours a day on the toilet in the act of voiding. This particularly applies to patients following spinal injury.

The value of intermittent catheterisation as a routine form of bladder management cannot be overemphasised. Education of medical and nursing personnel about the value of this technique is still required to overcome the many barriers that do exist to its use. Patients will take to intermittent catheterisation with ease provided they are properly counselled by clinicians or nursing staff committed to its use.

Sterile intermittent catheterisation (SIC)

This method of catheterisation is performed under aseptic conditions, usually by medical or nursing staff in the setting of a hospital or clinic. It is generally used for the management of inefficient bladder emptying in patients with neuropathic bladders or following surgery for stress incontinence (it is current practice in the United States to teach patients to use intermittent catheterisation after surgery for stress incontinence so that they may be discharged home early after surgery, continuing to use CISC until bladder emptying is efficient). On each occasion a catheter is passed using full aseptic principles. The catheter is discarded after a single use as is usual in a hospital setting.

SIC is correct in a hospital setting where resistant micro-organisms are present and cross-contamination is possible. However, the use of a sterile technique is inappropriate in everyday life, being too time-consuming and unnecessarily wasteful of resources. Therefore in the community, clean intermittent catheterisation is the norm.

Clean intermittent catheterisation (CIC)

This method, also known as clean intermittent self-catheterisation (CISC) (Lapides *et al.* 1972; Murray *et al.* 1984) is performed by the patient or by a care attendant, nurse or relative when the patient is unable to do this for him/herself. This technique is designed for patient use in an everyday setting. The patient is taught how to insert a fine-bore catheter into the bladder using a clean rather than sterile technique. It is important to emphasise to the patient that CISC is not harmful and that it may be performed five or six times a day without causing urethral injury if correctly used. A common misconception is that a disposable catheter should be used on each occasion. This is quite unnecessary and wasteful. A single plastic catheter of small calibre (10, 12 or 14 Ch) may be used over and over again and should be made to last for at least a week. Most patients may keep a catheter in use for four weeks. It is important to advise the patient to wash the catheter carefully after each use, store in a clean polythene bag in-between times, but not to immerse the catheter in antiseptic overnight (*Milton* is not recommended, since infection rates appear to be increased with this technique).

The patient is taught by a nurse trained in the technique. It may be necessary for the patient to use a mirror to guide catheter insertion in the first place. Once they become familiar with their anatomy, most patients manage catheterisation without difficulty by feel alone.

Pharmacological treatment of voiding disorders

Drugs which have been used to improve detrusor function include bethanecol chloride, distigmine bromide (Cameron 1966) and intravesical prostaglandin E2 and F2 (Bultitude *et al.* 1976; Delaere *et al.* 1981). These drugs have been widely used but recently appear to be losing popularity. The author's view is that none of these drugs have been conclusively shown to be of any long-term benefit and much of the published data are conflicting. It is important to realise that if the bladder does not contract, nothing will make it do so except perhaps direct nerve-root stimulation.

Alpha-adrenergic blocking agents are useful in males with urodynamically proven bladder neck obstruction. This condition is exceedingly rare in the female and thus these agents which include phenoxybenzamine, prazosin and indoramin find little place in the management of outflow obstruction in the female. The occasional patient who has a neurologically induced voiding disorder may have improved bladder emptying with alpha-adrenergic blockade.

Post-operative voiding problems may be improved by a small dose of an anxiolytic such as diazepam (Stanton and Cardozo 1979).

Surgical management

Urethral dilatation

If outflow obstruction is due to urethral stenosis, urethral dilatation will help to relieve the symptoms (Worth 1986). Provided there is adequate external sphincter function, a generous urethral dilatation with Hegars sounds may be performed without causing incontinence. Alternatively, an Otis urethrotome may be employed. Dilatation up to 45 Ch may be performed without causing incontinence in the normal female. It seems illogical to employ the cutting blade as it does not appear to contribute to the results and increases urethral bleeding and patient discomfort.

Urethral calibration is very rarely used nowadays for the assessment of urethral diameter (Farrar and Turner-Warwick 1979). Urethral obstruction is either stenotic or functional. If urethral stenosis is present, dilatation will help but will be likely to recur, as it does in the male, when healing of the dilated area occurs by scarring. Patient self-dilatation with a wide-bore catheter may be of use in these patients after initial surgical overdilatation. If urethral obstruction is functional, dilatation will provide a longer-lasting response and is helped if the primary cause of the problem is discovered and remedied.

Bladder neck incision

The place of bladder neck incision in the female with 'outflow obstruction' is a contentious issue. Bladder neck obstruction in the female is rare. Continence in some patients is often entirely or largely based upon a normally functioning bladder neck mechanism. Unless a diagnosis of bladder neck obstruction is confirmed by pressure/flow video-urodynamics, bladder neck incision *should never be performed.* The author has never seen a case of bladder neck obstruction.

Specific conditions

Asymptomatic voiding disorder

No active treatment is necessary if a voiding disorder is present without symptoms. If urinary tract infection occurs with residual urine, urethral dilatation may help; if not, daily intermittent catheterisation will remove the residual and reduce the incidence of infection. These patients should be investigated by urodynamic studies. An occasional patient with a neuropathic bladder condition may not complain of a voiding problem but has a thick-walled, high-pressure bladder with dilated upper urinary tracts.

Symptomatic voiding disorder

The treatment of each problem is according to the particular features that are provided by clinical investigation.

Acute retention of urine

The insertion of a small-calibre urethral catheter with drainage of the retained urine may be all that is necessary to permanently relieve this problem. Early intervention by catheterisation is highly recommended where acute retention presents. It is quite illogical to wait for a trial of drugs, hot baths, etc. as the single passage of a small urethral catheter will often relieve the problem in the majority of patients. Where the retention persists in spite of intermittent catheter drainage, the cause of the retention should be strenuously sought.

Chronic retention of urine

Some patients with chronic voiding disorders may never empty their bladders efficiently, always leaving residual urine. If the residual urine is under low pressure, does not produce infection or voiding symptoms then it may safely be left. No harm should come from the presence of asymptomatic residual urine. If problems arise as a result of residual urine, a regime of intermittent catheterisation should be introduced. Voiding efficiency does recover dramatically in many patients who have a surgical cause for their voiding difficulty (i.e. after surgery for stress incontinence). Their voiding pressures increase in response to the change in outflow resistance and residual urines almost invariably fall to nothing within a few days or weeks.

Those bladders that never recover normal function in spite of intermittent catheterisation are best managed with this technique indefinitely. Some clinicians do use either urethral dilatation or bladder neck incision for this condition but it is not considered appropriate in the author's view.

Rarely, a patient with chronic retention will not tolerate the regime of intermittent catheterisation (usually for psychological reasons). A surface urinary diversion may be the only option open for this patient.

Neurological disorders

Neurological disorders will either produce problems with bladder emptying or urinary incontinence or both. The urodynamic abnormality must be investigated with urodynamic study in all patients with a neurological aetiology. If failure of bladder emptying is the primary problem, intermittent catheterisation is the ideal. This form of management is dependent upon the ability and motivation of the patient or the presence of carers. If the patient is unable to self-catheterise or this form of management is socially unacceptable for many reasons, an in-dwelling catheter may be the last line of management. An in-dwelling urethral catheter that is chosen for long-term management should be of small calibre, changed regularly, positioned properly and have long-term medical supervision. All this is necessary to avoid the problems of catheter rejection, infection, stones and urethral destruction which are frequently caused by neglected catheter management. The solution in these patients with urethral destruction is surgical urethral closure and permanent suprapubic catheter drainage.

Conclusion

Listen to the symptoms in the female patient and voiding disorders will be detected early. They can then be treated appropriately. Acute retention should never be overlooked or trivialised. The patient is usually right. Surgical treatment of voiding disorders is usually the last resort after urodynamic investigation and conservative measures have been tried first.

References

Abrams, P.H. and Torrens, M. (1979) Urine flow studies. Symposium on Clinical Urodynamics. *Urol Clin North Am* **6**, 71–9

Barrett, D.M. (1978) Evaluation of psychogenic urinary retention. *J Urol* **120**, 191–2

Bollinger, B. and Mikkelesen, A.L. (1985) Leiomyoma of the urinary bladder. *Urol Int* **40**, 43–4

Bultitude, M.I., Hills, N.H. and Shuttleworth, K.E.D. (1976) Clinical and experimental studies on the action of prostaglandins and their synthesis inhibitors on detrusor muscle in vitro and in vivo. *Br J Urol* **48**, 631–7

Cameron, M.D. (1966) Distigmine Bromide (Ubretid) in the prevention of post-operative retention of urine. *J Obstet Br Commonwealth* **73**, 847–8

Coptcoat, M.J. and Shah, P.J.R. (1987) How does bladder function change in the early period after surgical alteration in outflow resistance? *J R Soc Med* **80**, 753–4

Cox, R. and Worth, P.H.L. (1986) Chronic retention after extratrigonal phenol injection for bladder instability. *Br J Urol* **58**, 229–30

Deane, A.M. and Worth, P.H.L. (1985) Female chronic urinary retention. *Br J Urol* **57**, 24–6

Delaere, K.P.J., Thomas, C.M.G., Moonen, W.A. and Debruyne, F.M.J. (1981) The value of intravesical prostaglandin E2 and F2 in women with abnormalities of bladder emptying. *Br J Urol* **53**, 306–9

Farrar, D. and Turner-Warwick, R.T. (1979) Outflow obstruction in the female. Symposium on Clinical Urodynamics. *Urol Clin North Am* **6**, 217–25

Fidas, A., Galloway, N.T.M., Varma, J. *et al.* (1987) Sacral reflex latency in acute retention in female patients. *Br J Urol* **59**, 311–13

Fox, M., Jarvis, G.J. and Henry, L. (1976) Idiopathic chronic urinary retention in the female. *Br J Urol* **47**, 797–803

Fraser, A.C. (1966) The late effects of Wertheim's hysterectomy on the urinary tract. *J Obstet Gynaecol Br Commonwealth* **73**, 1002–7

Giesy, J.D. (1986) Voiding problems in women. *Postgrad Med* **79**, 271–8

Guttmann, L. and Frankel, H. (1966) The value of intermittent catheterisation in the early management of traumatic paraplegia and tetraplegia. *Paraplegia* **4**, 63–84

Hemrika, D.J., Schutte, M.F. and Bleker, O.P. (1986) Elsberg syndrome: a neurologic basis for acute urinary retention in patients with genital herpes. *Obstet Gynecol* **68**, 37S–39S

Klarskov, P., Anderson, J.T., Asmussen, C.F. *et al.* (1987) Acute urinary retention in women: a prospective study of 18 consecutive cases. *Scand J Urol Nephrol* **21**, 29–31

Krane, R.J. and Siroky, M.B. (1900) Psychogenic voiding dysfunction. pp. 257–74

Lapides, J., Diokno, C., Silber, S.J. and Lowe, B.S. (1972) Clean, intermittent self-catheterisation in the treatment of urinary tract disease. *J Urol* **107**, 458–61

Lose, G., Jorgensen, L., Mortensen, S.O. *et al.* (1987) Voiding difficulties after colposuspension. *Obstet Gynecol* **69**, 33–8

Lyngdorf, P., Frimodt-Moller, C. and Jeppesen, N. (1986) Voiding disturbances following anal surgery. *Urol Int* **41**, 67–9

Murray, K., Lewis, P., Blannin, J. and Shepherd, A. (1984) Clean intermittent self-catheterisation in the management of adult lower urinary tract dysfunction. *Br J Urol* **56**, 379–80

Oates, J.K. and Greenhouse, P.R.D.H. (1978) Retention of urine in anogenital herpetic infection. *Lancet* 691–2

Preminger, G.M., Steinhardt, G.F., Mandell, J. *et al.* (1983) Acute urinary retention in female patients: diagnosis and treatment. *J Urol* **130**, 112–13

Ryttov, N., Aagaard, J. and Hertz, J. (1985) Retention of urine in genital herpetic infection. *Urol Int* **40**, 22–4

Shah, P.J.R., Whiteside, C.G., Milroy, E.J.G. and Turner-Warwick, R.T. (1981) Radiological assessment of the male bladder – a clinical and urodynamic assessment. *Br J Urol* **53**, 567–70

Shah, P.J.R., Whiteside, C.G., Milroy, E.J.G. and Turner-Warwick, R.T. (1983) The hypersensitive female urethra – a catheter diagnosis? *Proc XIIIth Annual Meeting of the International Continence Society*, pp. 202–3

Smith, P.H., Turnbull, G.A., Currie, D.W. and Peel, K.R. (1969) The urological complications of Wertheim's hysterectomy. *Br J Urol* **41**, 685–8

Stamey, T.A. (1973) Endoscopic suspension of the vesical neck for urinary incontinence. *Surg Gynecol Obstet* **136**, 547–54

Stanton, S.L. and Cardozo, L.D. (1979) A comparison of vaginal and suprapubic surgery in the correction of incontinence due to urethral sphincter incompetence. *Br J Urol* **51**, 497–9

Stanton, S.L., Ozsoy, C. and Hilton, P. (1983) Voiding difficulties in the female: prevalence, clinical and urodynamic review. *Obstet Gynecol* **61**, 144–7

Walter, S., Olesen, K.P., Hald, T. *et al.* (1982) Urodynamic evaluation after vaginal repair and colposuspension. *Br J Urol* **54**, 377–80

Worth, P.H.L. (1986) 'Urethrotomy' in S.L. Stanton and E.A. Tanagho (Eds) *Surgery for Female Incontinence* (2nd ed.), pp. 185–91. London and Berlin: Springer-Verlag

17

Post-operative voiding disorders

Timothy R. Sayer

Normal voiding appears to be a simple process but there are a number of complex factors which need to be co-ordinated to complete bladder emptying. Voiding is essentially a combination of bladder contraction and outlet relaxation to enable rapid and complete emptying. The neurological control of this mechanism is complex, hence any disturbance, either neurological or psychological, can affect voiding. Normal female voiding is rapid with relatively low intravesical pressures. Bladder contraction in females is of significantly lower pressure than the male and female voiding pressures may be low or even unrecordable in spite of rapid and effective voiding. Low recordable pressures occur because the detrusor contraction occurs with very low bladder resistance.

The bladder is an unreliable witness and nowhere more so is this apparent than in the history obtained of women with voiding disorders. Versi and Cardozo (1988) reported an incidence of spontaneous poor voiding in approximately 5–13% of perimenopausal women. Objectively voiding disorders occur in approximately 3–8% of the population.

Post-operative voiding difficulties may occur due to predisposing factors in women undergoing routine gynaecological surgery, or may occur following bladder neck surgery for stress incontinence of urine. Each of these areas will be considered separately.

Voiding problems after routine surgery

A good pre-operative history is important. Some 2–5% of women with a history of difficult voiding pre-operatively will develop post-operative retention. The common causes of poor voiding are shown in Table 17.1.

Neurological causes

Patients with a chronic neurological problem are more liable to develop post-operative voiding difficulties. Such patients are classically those with multiple sclerosis, transverse myelitis or those patients who have suffered previous cerebro-vascular accidents.

Pharmacological causes

Patients taking anti-cholinergic treatment, tricyclic antidepressants and sedatives are liable to difficulties in voiding post-surgery.

Table 17.1   Causes of female voiding difficulties

Neurological	Multiple sclerosis
	Diabetes mellitus
	Cerebrovascular accidents
Urological	Urinary tract infection
	Calculus
	Urethral diverticulum
	Urethral stricture
Drugs	Anticholinergic
	Antidepressant
Constipation	
Post-operative	Immobility/pain
	Hysterectomy
	Vaginal repair
	Bladder neck procedure for stress incontinence
	After any surgical procedure
Psychogenic	

Urological causes

Any inflammatory lesions of the lower urinary tract or of the genital tract will increase the risk of post-operative voiding difficulties. The urethral syndrome may lead to urethral stenosis and therefore post-operative voiding disorder.

Psychogenic causes

Urinary retention may develop in the absence of significant organic disease. Patients with psychogenic retention range from those with episodic acute retention to those who have learned to inhibit micturition (Barrett 1980).

The patient developing retention therefore should provide an MSSU to exclude urinary tract infection and should clearly be catheterised. If the patient has not had a bladder neck procedure performed then a urethral catheter should be inserted and drainage of the bladder obtained until diagnosis has been reached. Most patients will void spontaneously 48 hours following removal of the catheter.

If the patient suffers from long-term urological problems then suprapubic drainage is preferable.

Voiding difficulties after bladder neck surgery

In order to understand the aetiology of voiding disorders after bladder neck surgery the reasons for cure must be considered but these are unclear. Clearly, elevation of the bladder neck and an increase in urethral resistance are major factors. Anterior vaginal repair, colposuspension (Stanton and Cardozo 1979) and endoscopic bladder neck support (Coptcoat *et al.* 1987) have all been shown to increase urethral resistance. Lose *et al.* (1987) found that colposuspension may introduce an element of urethral obstruction which leads to a significant proportion of immediate as well as late voiding difficulties. In their study 25% of the patients developed severe voiding difficulties in the immediate post-operative course. Of particular importance to Lose was the fact that low pressure voiding, where the detrusor pressure was less than 15 cm of water pre-operatively, was found to predispose significantly to immediate post-operative voiding difficulties. Another 20% of his patients developed late voiding difficulties. He emphasised that pre-operative evaluation of both bladder and urethral function and the use of proper surgical technique are required to avoid voiding difficulties after colposuspension.

Hosker et al. (1991) described equally comparable success rates of bladder neck surgery where the bladder neck is supported only and not over-elevated. They studied 46 premenopausal stress incontinent women who underwent either Burch colposuspension or Aldridge fascial sling. Bladder neck surgery had a cure rate of between 85% and 90% in both groups which is comparable to that reported by other centres but no significant effect on voiding was demonstrated.

Even with pre-operative urodynamic assessment followed by careful surgical technique to try and minimise the risk of voiding disorders, some patients will inevitably develop voiding difficulties. All patients undergoing bladder neck procedures should have the suprapubic bladder drainage. A catheter specimen of urine should be examined during the post-operative recovery. Constipation should be avoided and the patient mobilised. If the patient continues to have problems following surgery then urodynamic investigation is easy to perform and may help elucidate an answer. Pharmacological stimulation of an underactive detrusor muscle can be tried in women with poor voiding but often gives poor results.

Two alternative forms of management are surgical or clean intermittent self-catheterisation. Surgical treatment involves urethral dilatation or Otis urethrotomy or endoscopic bladder neck incision. At all times care should be taken to avoid over-dilatation and to minimise the risk of reproducing sphincter weakness or incontinence. Otis urethrotomy serves the same purpose as a simple dilatation but incisions of the urethra produce significant bleeding, requiring the patient to be catheterised urethrally to enable this to settle. If surgery does not help the patient overcome voiding disorders then the technique of clean, intermittent self-catheterisation must be employed. Lapides et al. first developed this technique in 1972. Patients needing to perform this procedure need to be assessed and counselled as they need eyesight, manual dexterity and motivation to perform the procedure. There are many different forms of catheter. Significant bacteriuria can be expected in up to 40% of patients but in the absence of symptoms these patients do not require antibiotic therapy.

Summary

Voiding disorders cause much distress in women, particularly following bladder neck surgery and rapidly lead to lack of patient confidence. The anxiety which it generates forces further positive feedback leading to further episodes of retention. In order to minimise this all patients should have full pre-operative urodynamic assessment to assess the strength of detrusor contraction and to assess whether there is any evidence of increased outflow resistance in patients pre-operatively. All patients should be counselled as regards the possibility of long-term voiding disorders following bladder neck surgery and those at high risk of voiding disorder need counselling about clean intermittent self-catheterisation.

Surgical technique is important. Surgery for stress incontinence should aim to support the bladder neck and not to obstruct it.

References

Barrett, D.M. (1978) Evaluation of psychogenic urinary retention. *J Urol* **120**, 191–2

Coptcoat, M.J., Shah, P.J.R., Cumming, J. *et al.* (1987) How does bladder function change in the early period after surgical alteration in outflow resistance?: preliminary communication. *J R Soc Med* **80**, 753–4

Hosker, G.L., Sayer, T.R. and Warrell, D.W. (1991) Does successful abdominal bladder neck surgery alter voiding? *Neurourol Urodyn* **10**, 449–50

Lapides, J., Diokno, A.C., Silber, S.J. and Lowe, B.S. (1972) Clean intermittent self-catheterisation in the treatment of urinary tract disease. *J Urol* **107**, 458–61

Lose, G., Jorgensen, L., Mortensen, S.O. *et al.* (1987) Voiding difficulties after colposuspension. **69**, 33–7

Stanton, S.L. and Cardozo, L.D. (1979) Comparison of vaginal and suprapubic surgery in the correction of incontinence due to urethral sphincter incompetence. *J Urol* **51**, 497–9

Versi, E. and Cardozo, L.D. (1988) 'Oestrogens and lower urinary tract function' in J.W.W. Studd and M.I. Whitehead (Eds). *The Menopause*, pp. 76–84. Oxford: Blackwell Scientific

18

Faecal incontinence – should the obstetrician and gynaecologist be involved?

Clive Spence-Jones

Introduction

It is surprising that obstetricians and gynaecologists have little knowledge about faecal incontinence. There are few of us who, having witnessed extensive tears of the perineum, have not wondered how it will 'go back together', let alone function normally. Recent investigation of women in the puerperium using endoanal ultrasound suggests that damage to the anal sphincters occurs far more frequently than we realised. This damage causes immediate anorectal symptoms that are not reported by mothers unless asked. Furthermore, in women who present to coloproctologists with major anorectal incontinence, anal sphincter disruption and anal sphincter denervation are the characteristic findings. The incidence of faecal incontinence in patients with uterovaginal prolapse and urinary incontinence is higher than the general population, but this history is rarely elicited and an opportunity to combine surgical cure at the same operation is missed.

It is the responsibility of all those supervising childbirth to identify the events causing anal sphincter damage and to reduce these to a minimum. Poor control of bowel contents must be considered together with other symptoms including alteration of urinary control, dyspareunia, loss of muscle tone and perineal pain. It is no longer acceptable to regard such events as 'the inevitable sequelae of vaginal delivery'.

To understand the way in which obstetric events predispose to faecal incontinence it is necessary first to consider the factors involved in maintaining anal continence. The situations related to childbirth where the perineum and anal sphincters are at increased risk of damage are discussed together with the findings of recent studies using endoanal ultrasound.

Mechanism of anorectal continence

There are many parallels with theories of urinary continence. In addition to providing a reservoir capable of being emptied at a socially convenient time which is able to resist increases in intra-abdominal pressure, the anal canal differentiates flatus from stool and allows independent passage. The lower rectum and anal canal are normally empty. The flap valve theory of anorectal continence proposes that intra-abdominal forces are applied to a high pressure zone in the lower rectum thus occluding it and preventing passage of rectal contents into the anal canal. Parks popularised this theory and emphasised the importance of an acute anorectal angle created by the activity of the puborectalis muscle sling (innervation from direct branch of S_3 S_4 motor roots via the visceral surface of the pelvic diaphragm). Recent studies showing higher pressure in the anal canal, caudal to the rectum, have questioned the validity of this theory (Bartolo *et al.* 1986). The internal anal sphincter (continuation of the circular smooth muscle of the rectum) is in a continuous state of contraction and accounts for 70–80% of the resting anal pressure. The external anal sphincter, innervated by the pudendal nerve (S_2 S_3), shows tonic activity and is under voluntary control. Together with intact sensory innervation, the anal sphincter complex plays the major role in maintaining anorectal continence.

Incidence of faecal incontinence

There is no objective way of evaluating women with anorectal incontinence (i.e. no equivalent to the ICS pad test for urinary incontinence) to assess the type of loss – symptoms are grouped on clinical features.

1 Faecal staining – often due to local perianal conditions, e.g. prolapsing haemorrhoids.
2 Incontinence of flatus – most frequently a reflection of reduced internal anal sphincter function.
3 Incontinence of loose stool – may be a normal response to prolific diarrhoea.
4 Incontinence of solid stool – combination of structural alteration of the internal and external anal sphincter often combined with denervation.

Patients may also report urgency which is defined as an inability to delay defecation for more than five minutes and is a symptom of reduced external anal sphincter function.

The true incidence of faecal incontinence is not known but there is an increase in the fifth and sixth decade, with a ratio of approximately 8:1 women to men. In North American literature, in women presenting with faecal incontinence, non-obstetric causes (e.g. previous anorectal surgery for sepsis) account for approximately 40% of patients. In the UK, slightly more are attributed to non-obstetric causes, approximately 60%. In a series of 62 women with faecal incontinence due to obstetric trauma where internal anal sphincter defects were not suspected, 90% were identified by endoanal ultrasound as having an external anal sphincter defect, 65% had an internal sphincter defect and 57% had evidence of pudendal neuropathy (Burnett *et al.* 1991).

In gynaecology patients with urinary incontinence or prolapse, a history of faecal incontinence is identified in 4% of women (Spence-Jones *et al.* 1994). This is considerably more than the incidence in the general population of 0.5–1.0%. Failure to obtain a history of anorectal symptoms may miss the opportunity to combine surgical cure of co-existent pelvic floor disorders. Additionally, it is worth noting that 10% of women presenting with faecal incontinence to a coloproctologist will have a significant problem with stress urinary incontinence.

Incidence of faecal incontinence after vaginal delivery

There are no long-term follow-up studies of anorectal function after vaginal delivery – the Oxford Perinatal Database does not list these problems under a separate

Table 18.1   Incidence of faecal incontinence after vaginal delivery

	Incontinence solid/liquid	Incontinence of flatus	Follow-up
Snooks 1986	2/102	Not stated	2 months
Cornes 1990	2/101	13/101	6 months
Sultan 1993a	6/127	6/127	6 months
NCT Survey 1993	Not stated	500/2000	Not stated

section. The studies which consider anorectal symptoms in women after vaginal delivery are listed in Table 18.1.

Unlike urinary incontinence these symptoms are rarely noticed antenatally and a significant proportion will recover without specific treatment in the first three months after delivery. In the studies which also identified women with stress urinary incontinence, it was noticed that there was no relationship between the symptoms, implying different aetiology for impairment of urinary and faecal control postpartum. However, it may be that, later in life, the effect of denervation becomes more significant, allowing funtional disruption of urinary and bowel control (Laurberg and Swash 1989).

Denervation

Investigation of women with major faecal incontinence frequently identifies evidence of denervation of the external anal sphincter/puborectalis (Snooks and Henry 1985), together with reduced sensory perception in the anal canal. The causes of denervation are damage to the pudendal nerve during chronic straining/constipation, and damage during childbirth. Denervation in pelvic muscles is identified by characteristic changes seen in the histology of biopsies, EMG, and measurement of the pudendal nerve terminal conduction latency, which is prolonged when large myelinated fibres are absent. Studies on women in the postnatal period do not agree on the highest risk factors for denervation. Allen *et al.* (1990) identified EMG evidence of puborectalis reinnervation in 80% of primiparous women, there was increased denervation with large babies and long second stage of labour including evidence of pelvic floor denervation in women delivered by LSCS in the second stage of labour. Snooks *et al.* (1984, 1990) however, identified multiparous women delivered by forceps as most likely to show evidence of denervation of the external anal sphincter. In 60–70% of women with evidence of denervation, there is significant recovery of the function in the pudendal nerve during the first three months after delivery.

Cornes *et al.* (1991) identified evidence of reduced anal canal sensory awareness to electrical stimulation after vaginal delivery but this recovered within six months in all patients except those with a third degree tear.

A long history of constipation, starting after having children, may contribute to the process of denervation and has been identified in women who present with uterovaginal prolapse (Spence-Jones *et al.* 1994).

Anal sphincter disruption

Complete disruption of the external anal sphincter, with or without denervation, is often identified in women with major faecal incontinence. External anal sphincter disruption is amenable to primary or secondary repair but repair is not successful in women with associated denervation. Until the use of endoanal ultrasound, identification of defects has conventionally been by clinical examination – seeing a tear at the time of perineal trauma or feeling a defect some months later. Additionally, EMG 'mapping' gives evidence of areas with reduced striated muscle but the technique is painful, because of multiple needle insertions. Reduced anal voluntary contraction pressures, in the absence of evidence of denervation, is seen in women with external anal sphincter defects but is not sensitive or specific.

Disruption of the internal anal sphincter can be identified at the time of trauma. Once healing has taken place, however, until endoanal ultrasound was introduced, defects could only be implied by the finding of a low resting anal pressure. There are no surgical techniques available to effect successful secondary repair of the internal anal sphincter.

In the last five years anal endosonography has been introduced. Using a rotating rectal probe, a 7 MHz transducer (focal range 2–4.5 cm) contained in a sonolucent plastic cone, the internal and external anal sphincters can be visualised. The technique produces images of the upper middle and lower anal canal and the appearance of the images has been extensively validated (see Figures 18.1 and 18.2). In a study of 150 women before and after delivery, of whom, 79 were primiparous, incontinence of flatus or faecal urgency were identified in 13% of the primiparous women and 23% of the multiparous women. Anal endosonography identified anal sphincter defects in 35% of the primiparous women and 40% of the multiparous women (Sultan *et al.* 1993a). Internal anal sphincter defects were associated with a lower resting anal pressure and external anal sphincter defects were associated with lower voluntary contraction pressure. Only 30% of the women with sphincter defects identified on ultrasound had bowel symptoms, and the symptoms had resolved in 30% of these women by six months' postpartum. Multivariate analysis showed that forceps delivery was the single independent factor associated with the development of internal and external anal sphincter defects. The implication from this study is that anal sphincter damage occurs more frequently than is recognised by those doing the perineal suturing at the time of delivery, and that in some of these mothers it is associated with minor anorectal symptoms.

In the future, studies of the pelvic floor using MRI may well provide additional information about changes in the puborectalis/levator ani muscle (Aronson 1990). Anecdotal reports of severe unilateral damage from traumatic vaginal delivery imply that the information from MRI will be very valuable.

Risk factors for anal sphincter disruption

Episiotomy

Traditional teaching is that episiotomy reduces perineal trauma and expedites vaginal delivery. Studies to investigate these claims have mostly been observational, and only two randomised controlled trials are available comparing liberal and restrictive

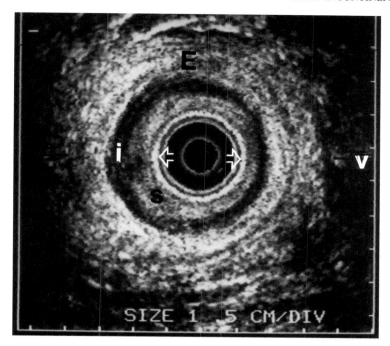

Figure 18.1   Normal anal endosonographic appearance of the mid-anal canal in a 27-year-old female. Anterior, is to the right of the image. The arrows indicate the bright double ring reflection from the probe within the anal canal.
V = vagina
S = subepithelium
i = internal anal sphincter
E = external anal sphincter

use of episiotomy in spontaneous vaginal deliveries. There are no studies which document the incidence of faecal incontinence or other anorectal symptoms in relationship to a particular episiotomy practice. Isager-Sally *et al.* (1986) reported the incidence of flatus incontinence in 900 women who had an episiotomy, and were randomised to three different types of repair. Flatus incontinence was reported in 13–20% of mothers at three months' postpartum.

Trauma is evaluated subjectively at the time of delivery by recording third and fourth degree tears. Sleep (Sleep *et al.* 1984; Sleep and Grant 1987) randomised 1000 women to two groups, liberal and restricted use of episiotomy; an episiotomy rate of 10% and 51% respectively were observed. The authors concluded that there was little support for liberal use of episiotomy to protect the perineum. A French National Survey noted that despite an increase in the episiotomy rate from 8.15% to 32.1% from 1972 to 1981, the incidence of third degree tears did not change.

Mediolateral episiotomy is associated with 0.1–1.8% third and fourth degree tears (Thacker and Banta 1983), whereas the risk of similar tears using midline episiotomy (standard practice throughout North America) is up to 13% (Coates *et al.* 1980; Shiono *et al.* 1990). It seems that a mediolateral episiotomy rate of approximately 20% is the standard to aim for in primiparous women predominantly for 'fetal

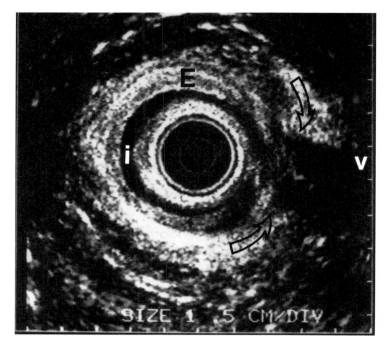

Figure 18.2 Anal endosonographic image taken from a 28-year-old female who had a 'repaired' third degree tear three months previously*. There is a persistent defect in the external anal sphincter (between open arrows).
* This woman complained of faecal urgency and flatus incontinence since delivery.

indications' (Harrison *et al.* 1984); below this rate there is an increased risk of spontaneous tears involving the anal sphincter, and significantly above this level there are extensions into the sphincter. The practice of midline episiotomy should not be encouraged as it is associated with three times more likely extension to the anal sphincters.

Operative vaginal delivery

Operative vaginal delivery poses the greatest threat to the perineum. Debates about the relative merits of forceps or ventouse have evaluated fetal outcome and maternal trauma. The Oxford Perinatal Database identifies standard and special indications for operative delivery (Vacca 1990). This excellent review identifies five controlled studies comparing vacuum extraction and forceps delivery. Significant maternal injury was reported in three of the five studies and was statistically more common in women allocated to forceps delivery (Odds ratio 0.38, 95% CI). In addition vacuum delivery was associated with less pain and less need for regional or general analgesia.

In a further randomised study, Johanson *et al.* (1993) compared delivery by forceps with delivery by vacuum extractor, where a new vacuum extractor policy was employed which dictated the cup to be used in specific situations. In the 296 women

Table 18.2 Functional results of repaired anal sphincter rupture up to one year postpartum

	Third degree	Incontinence solid/liquid	Incontinence of flatus
Haadem 1990	0.79%	9/21	1/21
Sorensen 1993	0.7%	9/38	5/38
Nielsen 1992	?	3/24	4/24
Sultan 1994	0.6%	3/34	11/34
Crawford 1993	4%	2/35	6/35
		26/152 (17%)	27/152 (18%)

allocated to vacuum extractor, there were 5% who suffered anal sphincter damage compared with 8% in the 311 women delivered by forceps – this difference was not significant. If vaginal tears to the fornix were included the respective figure became 11% and 17%, which was significant. There appeared to be no increased risk to the fetus from the different instruments, but the authors stated a need for a large randomised controlled trial to detect differences in rare events of serious fetal morbidity. The rate of maternal injury to mothers not randomised (218 forceps and 146 vacuum extractor in the time period of the study) was not stated.

Endoanal ultrasound has not been used to investigate the anal sphincters in a randomised study of vacuum and forceps delivery. An observational study of operative vaginal delivery (17 delivered by vacuum extraction; 26 using forceps), identified anal sphincter defects in 21/26 (81%) of the forceps deliveries. In only one of the 26 patients had a third degree tear been identified at the time of delivery. In the vacuum extraction patients, anal sphincter tears were identified in 21% and in none of these women was anal sphincter damage identified at the time of delivery. Symptoms of incontinence (flatus plus liquid stool) were identified in 38% of the women delivered by forceps and in 12% of the vacuum extraction group. Only two (4%) of the control group had defecatory symptoms (Sultan *et al.* 1993b). Clearly this study needs to be repeated with deliveries randomised to vacuum or forceps.

Third degree tears

The terms third and fourth degree tear are used to describe trauma to the anal sphincter with or without anal canal mucosa involvement. The definitions are interpreted vaguely, but the following classification is simple and if universally adopted would make interpretation of the data easier (see Figure 18.2).

1 First degree: laceration of the vaginal epithelium or perineal skin only.
2 Second degree: involvement of the perineal muscles but not the anal sphincters.
3 Third degree: disruption of the anal sphincter muscles which may be partial or complete without involvement of the anal epithelium.
4 Fourth degree: a third degree tear with disruption of the anal epithelium as well.

An isolated tear of the anorectal epithelium without involvment of the anal sphincters (buttonhole) is rare and should be classified as a separate event.

There is a widely held belief that identification of sphincter trauma at the time of delivery with primary repair, causes minimal long-term sequelae. Recent research has shown that unfortunately this is not true (see Table 18.2).

Third and fourth degree tears are most frequently identified in nulliparous women. It is rare to have severe lacerations in a multiparous woman unless the delivery is complicated by a large baby/shoulder dystocia.

Two studies have examined the endoscopic appearance of the anal sphincters after primary repair of third or fourth degree tears. Neilsen *et al.* (1992) examined 24 patients 12 months after delivery. All patients were thought to have had a satisfactory primary repair by the obstetrician. Endoscopy was normal in 10/24 patients. There was a defect of the external anal sphincter in 13 patients and an isolated defect of internal anal sphincter in one patient (this was the only internal anal sphincter defect identified). No patients had symptoms of incontinence if the sphincters were intact on the ultrasound.

Sultan *et al.* (1994) studied 34 women who had sustained third or fourth degree tear sutured by the obstetric registrar or senior registrar. Anal endosonography showed sphincter defects in 29/34 (85%) of these women. In one patient the internal sphincter alone was deficient, in five the external sphincter alone and in the remainder both anal sphincters showed defects. Wound infection occurred in six patients but there was no association between this and the integrity of the sphincters on ultrasound. Symptoms of anal incontinence are shown in Table 18.2. The study was not randomised but was compared with the remaining 8553 deliveries in the period of the study. Forceps delivery, birth weight >4 kg, and occipitoposterior position at delivery were all significantly more common in women who sustained a third degree tear.

Advice about the type of delivery recommended for subsequent delivery of women who sustained a third or fourth degree tear with their first baby is difficult. Bek and Laurberg (1992) reported the outcome of 121 women in this situation. In the 56 women who had a subsequent vaginal delivery, 23 (41%) had experienced transient, and 7% permanent, anal incontinence. Of the 23 women who had transient incontinence after their first delivery, 17% developed permanent anal incontinence after subsequent vaginal delivery.

What is the role of physiotherapy? Antenatal advice may help reduce the postnatal problems but this has not been adequately demonstrated. Postnatal advice about pelvic floor exercises is universally given but it is time-consuming and may well not be appropriate for all women. This is an area where the beneficial effects will rely heavily on the enthusiasm of the individual physiotherapist.

Conclusion

Anorectal trauma at the time of vaginal delivery frequently causes sphincter damage that is recognised on endoanal ultrasound. This is associated with symptoms of faecal urgency and incontinence in some women. It may be that symptoms of incontinence will become more of a problem in women with sphincter defects with advancing age.

Requests for elective Caesarean section for no reason other than to avoid the possible trauma of a vaginal delivery are becoming more frequent. This is not the right way forward. As already described, at least 60% of women have no long-term effects on urinary control and only a few women are symptomatic of poor control of bowel function (although as many as 30% have evidence of anal sphincter damage on anal ultrasound). The challenge for us is to identify the women at high risk of long-term pelvic floor problems and offer them elective LSCS. It is clear that the majority of women with problems suffer the greatest damage at the time of their first baby, so it is no good shutting the door after the horse has bolted – we need to avoid trauma at the first delivery.

Training in the identification of anal sphincter damage at the time of delivery and evaluation of different approaches to the repair are areas where there is potential for significant reduction in maternal morbidity. It may be necessary to involve surgeons experienced in operations on the anal sphincter using techniques such as overlapping. The primary repair of the internal anal sphincter must be considered and evaluated with post-operative anal ultrasound.

The skill of obstetricians in the 1990s will not only be judged by achieving vaginal delivery with satisfactory outcome for the baby – we must also be confident that maternal pelvic floor function is preserved.

References

Allen, R.E., Hosker, G.L., Smith, A.R.B. and Warrell, D.W. (1990) Pelvic floor damage and childbirth: a neurophysiological study. *Br J Obstet Gynaecol* **97**, 770–9

Aronson, M.P., Lee, R.A. and Berquist, T.H. (1990) Anatomy of anal sphincters and related structures in continent women studied with magnetic resonance imaging. *Obstet Gynecol* **76**, 846–51

Bartolo, D.C.C., Roe, A.M., Locke-Edmunds, J.C. *et al.* (1986) Flap-valve theory of anorectal continence. *Br J Surg* **73**, 1012–4

Bek, K.M. and Laurberg, S. (1992) Risks of anal incontinence from subsequent vaginal delivery after a complete obstetric anal sphincter tear. *Br J Obstet Gynaecol* **99**, 724–6

Burnett, S.J.D. Spence-Jones, C., Speakman, T.M. *et al.* (1991) Unsuspected sphincter damage following childbirth revealed by anal endosonography. *Br J Radiology* **64**, 225–7

Coats, P.M., Chan, K.K., Wilkins, M. and Beard, R.J. (1980) A comparison between midline and mediolateral episiotomies. *Br J Obstet Gynaecol* **87**, 408–12

Cornes, H., Bartolo, D.C.C. and Stirrat, G.M. (1991) Changes in anal canal sensation after childbirth. *Br J Surg* **78**, 7477

Crawford, L.A., Quint, E.H., Pearl, M.L. and De Lancey, J.O.L. (1993) Incontinence following rupture of the anal sphincter during delivery. *Obstet Gynaecol* **82**, 527–31

Haadem, K., Dahlstrom, J.A. and Lingman, G. (1990) Anal sphincter function after delivery: a prospective study in women with sphincter rupture and controls. *Eur J Obstet Gynaecol Reprod Biol* **35**, 7–13

Harrison, R.F., Brennan, M., North, P.M. *et al.* (1984) Is routine episiotomy necessary? *Br J Med* **288**, 1971–5

Isager-Sally, L., Legarth, J., Jacobsen, B. and Bostofte, E. (1986) Episiotomy repair – immediate and long-term sequelae. A prospective randomized study of three different methods of repair. *Br J Obstet Gynaecol* **93**, 420–5

Johanson, R.B., Rice, C., Doyle, M. *et al.* (1993) A randomised prospective study comparing the new vacuum extractor policy with forceps delivery. *Br J Obstet Gynaecol* **100**, 524–30

Laurberg, S. and Swash, M. (1989) Effects of aging on the anorectal sphincters and their innervation. *Dis Colon Rectum* 737–42

Neilson, M.B., Hauge, C., Rasmussen, O.O. *et al.* (1992) Anal endosonographic findings in the follow-up of primarily sutured sphincteric ruptures. *Br J Surg* **79**, 104–6

Shiono, P., Klebanoff, M.A. and Carey, J.C. (1990) Midline episiotomies: more harm than good? *Obstet Gynaecol* **75**, 765–9

Sleep, J. and Grant, A. (1987) West Berkshire perineal management trial: three year follow up. *BMJ* **295**, 749–51

Sleep, J., Grant, A., Garcia, J. *et al.* (1984) West Berkshire perineal management trial. *BMJ* **289**, 587–90

Snooks, S.J., Setchell, M., Swash, M. and Henry, M.M. (1984) Injury to innervation of pelvic floor sphincter musculature in childbirth. *Lancet* 546–50

Snooks, S.J. and Henry, M.M. (1985) Faecal incontinence due to external anal sphincter division in childbirth is associated with damage to the innervation of the pelvic floor musculature: a double pathology. *Br J Obstet Gynaecol* **92**, 824–8

Snooks, S.J., Swash, M., Henry, M.M. and Setchell, M.E. (1986) Risk factors in childbirth causing damage to the pelvic floor innervation. *Int J Colorectal Dis* **1**, 20–4

Snooks, S.J., Swash, M., Mathers, S.E. and Henry, M.M. (1990) Effect of vaginal delivery on the pelvic floor: a 5-year follow-up. *Br J Surg* **77**, 1358–60

Sorenson S.M., Dondesen, H., Istre, O. and Vilmann, P. (1988) Perineal rupture following vaginal delivery – long term consequences. *Acta Obstet Gynaecol Scand* **67**, 315–18

Sprensen, M., Tetzschner, T., Rasmussen, O.O. *et al.* (1993) Sphincter rupture in childbirth. *Br J Surg* **80**, 392–4

Spence-Jones, C., Kamm, M.A., Henry, M.M. and Hudson, C.N. (1994) Bowel dysfunction: a pathogenic factor in uterovaginal prolapse and urinary stress incontinence. *Br J Obstet Gynaecol* **101**, 147–52

Sultan, A.H., Kamm, M.A., Bartram, C.I. and Hudson, C.N. (1993) Anal sphincter trauma during instrumental delivery. *Int J Gynaecol Obstet* **43**, 263–70

Sultan, A.H., Kamm, M.A., Hudson, C.N. *et al.* (1993) Anal-sphincter disruption during vaginal delivery. *N Engl J Med* **329**, 1905–11

Sultan, A.H., Kamm, M.A., Hudson, C.N. and Bartam, C.I. (1994) Third degree obstetric anal sphincter tears: risk factors and outcome of primary repair. *BMJ* **308**, 887–91

Thacker, S.B. and Banta, H.D. (1983) Benefits and risks of episiotomy: an interpretative review of the English language literature 1860–1980. *Obstet Gynecol Surv* **38**, 322–37

Vacca, A. and Keirse, M.J.N.C. (1990) 'Instrumental vaginal delivery' in I. Chalmers, M. Enkin and M.J.N.C. Keirse (Eds) *Effective Care in Pregnancy and Childbirth*, pp. 1216–33. Oxford: Oxford University Press

19

Basic investigations and treatment of faecal incontinence

Ed Kiff

People do not have a vocabulary for describing defaecation and therefore will not tell you about faecal incontinence. You will have to ask them. People put up with faecal incontinence for years, gradually confining their lives around the problem rather than confess. It will be kept a secret very often from their partners and best friends. The following simple questions should be put to all patients who you think might be at risk.

Urgency

When you get the feeling of wanting to move your bowels, do you have to rush to get to the lavatory? Would you get caught out on the way?

If the answer is yes then the patient either has a normal sphincter which has been overcome by diarrhoea or a weak voluntary sphincter.

Stool consistency

Is the motion solid or loose? Is it much more difficult to contain when loose or diarrhoea stool?

If the patient is incontinent of solid stool, then the sphincter is very weak indeed.

Prolapse

When you move your bowels do you feel part of your insides coming out and if so what size is it?

A grape-like swelling could well be mucosal prolapse or piles. If it is the size of a tomato or larger, this is a rectal prolapse. Incontinence is inevitable with rectal prolapse but the treatment is to fix the prolapse, rather than deal with the sphincters.

Difficulty wiping clean

Difficulty wiping clean is either due to mucosal prolapse or due to low resting pressure in the anus, usually due to a weakened internal sphincter.

Leakage

Do you leak during the rest of the day?

In the absence of a prolapse this is an index of resting pressure and therefore mainly internal sphincter activity. The most difficult thing to contain would be flatus and thereafter mucus and finally solid stool.

Examination

Having taken a history one has a good idea of what to expect. Examination will confirm many of these suspicions. With the patient in the left lateral position, look! Is there a loss of tissue between the anus and the introitus? This suggests an anterior sphincter weakness. Are there scars or fistulae? Does the anus gape on traction, if so the resting pressure and therefore internal sphincter is reduced. When the patient strains hard is there any prolapse or perineal descent? When the pelvic floor is generally weak, raised intra-abdominal pressure just bulges it out. This will interfere with the process of defaecation as well as continence. It is not unusual also to see a cystocele or uterine prolapse.

Next, feel. Feel the length of the canal. This will be reduced with perineal descent. The shorter the canal, the shorter is the high pressure zone and so the more likely is incontinence. Are there any gaps in the sphincter ring, particularly anteriorly? Is the ano–rectal angle normal or has it been flattened out due to a loss of tone in the puborectalis sling. Ask the patient to squeeze tight. You should feel puborectalis and an accentuation of the ano–rectal angle. If not there is most probably a neuropathy accounting for the pelvic floor muscle weakness. Examination would then be followed up by sigmoidoscopy particularly to exclude a proctitis or tumour and then either barium enema or colonoscopy as indicated.

Ano–rectal physiology studies

Ano–rectal manometry is simple and informative. We use a small water-filled balloon connected to a transducer and chart recorder but air-filled balloons and perfused catheters are also used. Using a station pull-through technique, measurement of maximal resting pressure and maximal voluntary contraction pressure is made. Seventy per cent or so of resting pressure is due to the internal sphincter activity and it is the best guide to its performance. The other 30% is due to resting activity in the voluntary muscles. Clearly all of the voluntary contraction pressure is due to voluntary muscles, particularly the external anal sphincter. Manometric findings may relate to symptoms and the underlying muscle weakness although it is not always quite so clear-cut. Some groups are now exploring the use of ambulatory anal pressure monitoring, particularly to look at the change in internal sphincter function with time.

There are many electro-physiological methods of investigation. Essentially what one wants to know is whether or not there is a neuropathy. Pudendal nerve terminal motor latency measurement is the gold standard. Prolonged latency occurs when the majority of fast acting neurones in the terminal portion of the pudendal nerve are lost. This is found in about 60% of patients presenting with neuropathic faecal incontinence. EMG studies which are painful and more complicated to perform will pick up neuropathy at an earlier stage. Measure of anal canal electro-mucosal sensitivity is a successful method of indirectly demonstrating pudendal neuropathy where the patient's awareness of increasing electrical discharges in the anal canal is measured. It is very likely that many other nerves supplying this area of the perineum are also damaged by the same process which gives rise to pudendal neuropathy. We know that there is a slow but definite deterioration of the neuropathy with time.

Ultrasound

Transanal ultrasonography has been developed in recent years and provides pictures of the sphincter muscles which has led to a better understanding of sphincter disruption particularly after childbirth and surgical intervention. It is probable that we have missed the disruption in some patients who have both disruption and neuropathy. This may be particularly pertinent to obstetricians who could use this investigation as part of their follow-up of mothers.

Treatment

Conservative

Having ruled out bowel diseases, there is no doubt that the most useful treatment and the essential first step is to thicken the stool wherever possible. This can be done by increasing the bulk in the diet either with bran or bulking agents such as Fybogel or Normacol or using agents such as loperamide or codeine. A small dose of loperamide used intermittently can have a tremendous benefit, allowing many patients who have previously been confined to the house to get out. If the patient already has a formed stool and yet is incontinent, this means that their sphincters are very weak and are likely to require surgery. Although I advise all patients to do pelvic floor exercises, it is likely only to be of significant benefit to those with a reasonable muscle bulk that is active on voluntary contraction and who can contain a solid stool. We have found some improvement in a subgroup of patients with the use of electrical stimulation of the sphincter but again there needs to be sufficient muscle bulk for this to be effective.

Surgical

Patients with incontinence who have a rectal prolapse are best treated by rectopexy. In most cases this would cure the incontinence although they may be left with some leakage due to internal sphincter weakness for a while. Less than 10% will require sphincter surgery subsequently. Patients with a defect in the sphincter ring, usually anterior, will require a sphincter repair. The aim here is to identify the muscle ends, without damaging the nerve supply which comes in posterolaterally, to produce an overlapping repair. In an anterior sphincter repair in a woman, I would continue this further upwards as a posterior colporrhaphy in order to gain good sphincter length. These patients do not require a colostomy. For sphincter repair following previous surgery such as fistula or trauma, colostomy is essential.

Most patients presenting with faecal incontinence have a pudendal neuropathy which leads to a loss of the ano–rectal angle. The operation of post-anal repair was designed to re-create this angle by suturing the limbs of the puborectalis sling within the intersphincteric space. However, the post-operative results do not correlate with the angle formed. Nonetheless, one would expect to get some 60–70% of patients continent after a post-anal repair. The operation is performed either in the jacknife position through a posterior sagittal approach or, more conventionally, in lithotomy. The intersphincteric space is entered posteriorly and the sling of puborectalis and then external anal sphincter are drawn together with a non-absorbable suture.

Wrapping muscle around the anal canal, particularly using grascilis, has been used for many years but has been of more interest lately due to the simultaneous implantation of a stimulator to create a neosphincter. The longer term results of this procedure are awaited, in particular to see if the addition of a stimulator contributes anything extra. It is possible that all of these procedures have worked by lengthening the anal canal and producing an angle. The aim of the stimulator is to convert the wrapped muscle from fast to slow twitch fibres.

There have been several attempts at implanting a mechanical sphincter but none are particularly successful.

Finally, there will be some patients whose pelvic floor and sphincter is so weak that they can neither defaecate adequately nor maintain continence. Some of these are best treated by having a colostomy. Similarly this is an effective treatment for patients who have failed other forms of surgery. The slight disadvantage of the colostomy and its bag is nothing compared to the misery of faecal incontinence.

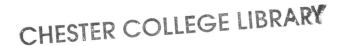